D0345402

Old-Fashioned Health Remedies That Work Best

Old-Fashioned Health Remedies That Work Best

Low cost natural time-tested
health boosters you can use
at home for successful self-care

L. L. SCHNEIDER, D.C., N.D.

in Association with

ROBERT B. STONE

Illustrations by GREG J. SCHNEIDER

PARKER PUBLISHING COMPANY, INC.

West Nyack, N.Y.

This book is a reference work based on research by the author. The opinions expressed herein are not necessarily those of or endorsed by the publisher. The directions stated in this book are in no way to be considered as a substitute for consultation with a duly licensed doctor.

Library of Congress Cataloging in Publication Data

Schneider, L L
Old-fashioned health remedies that work best.

1. Naturopathy. 2. Hygiene. I. Stone, Robert B., joint author. II. Title.
RZ440.S35 615'.535 76-56734
ISBN 0-13-633701-5

Printed in the United States of America

WHAT THIS BOOK CAN DO FOR YOU

Nature cures. Doctors are nature's helpers, but doctors are the first to admit it is nature that actually does the healing.

Modern man, however, has placed walls between himself and nature. The walls of houses, cars, subways, stores, and offices. His separation from nature has deprived him of many natural cures.

Did you know that nature has equipped the soles of our feet with a body-wide curative system? A network of nerves there provides the equivalent of a therapeutic massage wherever needed. But we separate ourselves from this natural healing with thick leather soles.

Did you know that nature has an herb, fruit, or vegetable containing the perfect ingredient for practically every internal weakness that affects us? Grazing animals are attracted to the kinds of growing things they need. Even dogs will eat grass when their body requires it. But man has separated himself from growing things and the yen or craving that is often nature's voice calling for help is automatically translated into pizza or apple pie patterns of modern eating.

This book gives nature a public address system. It calls out to you loud and clear what nature may have been trying to tell you in her own subtle way, but which has not gotten through to you.

As a result you may have less energy or you may be a grouch to your family or you may suffer a skin problem or pains and aches or the "miseries."

This book is full of nature's own first aid. It is not meant to replace your doctor. As the label says, "If pain persists, see your doctor." If your problem persists, by all means consult your local physician or health care specialist — he is an even better nature's helper than this book.

Preventive care is ignored by most of us in today's fast pace. When something goes wrong, then we pay attention. Nature gives us subtle signs that tip us off to save us pain and grief ahead of time. Simple steps are offered by nature to prevent many pains from turning from passing to permanent. If postponed, corrective steps can become more complicated and even drastic.

It's really all as simple as an apple a day. It might be beet juice, or the special use of a clothespin, or a massage you never knew about, or a short walk on gravel, or words to repeat to erase a memory pattern that is causing body tension, or an herb to use, an exercise to do.

Health is a natural state. On the pages ahead are scores of nature's remedies the author has tested in his practice (the names of patients in case histories have been changed, of course) and found to be amazingly effective. Many are easy to find close by. Some might take a trip to the country. All are low in cost, high in the relief and power for health they can bring. And I have never asked anyone to try a remedy which I would not use myself.

L. L. Schneider, D.C., N.D.

Acknowledgments

First of all, I dedicate this book to my wife, Joan. Without her many, many hours of diligent work, this book would not have been written. Throughout the years she has had the patience of Job and understanding to give me the strength and encouragement needed while I have been so involved with my practice.

I also dedicate this book to our sons, Greg and Kent, who have lent their support and encouragement by using these natural remedies to the advantage of their own better health. Greg has kindly contributed his talent in producing the illustrations for this book.

To my patients of the past, present, and future. I dedicate this book, for these people have had faith and the belief that these recommendations would help. This belief is the connecting link that has created the miracle, for it has been said, "As a man thinketh in his heart, so is he."

My very special thanks go to Mr. Robert B. Stone for his foresight in recognizing the value of old-fashioned health remedies, thereby investing his time and skill.

Also, my special thanks to Dr. Jack Schwarz for pointing out my abilities, which we all have if only someone will take the time to encourage us to pursue the things we sometimes doubt we have the ability to do.

CONTENTS

1

OLD FASHIONED HEALTH REMEDIES ARE WINNING NEW RESPECT TODAY

When I was a boy, every family had its own "resident physician" — in my family it was my grandmother.

She always had the right remedy — a poultice, a compress, a special soup, a certain juice. I had a great respect for my grandmother's home remedies. My mother learned a lot from her, too.

Today I am a doctor. And I have even greater respect for these home remedies.

Doctors seldom make house calls any more. Many patients phone for advice. Believe me, I do not tell my patients to take two aspirin and phone me in the morning. Instead, I tell many to try a particular old-fashioned health remedy. Some work so well and so fast, they don't have to phone me the next morning. They have recovered and forgotten about their problem.

I am talking about relieving and alleviating such conditions as:

- Stomach distress
- Headaches
- Back trouble
- Colds and sinus
- Cuts and sores
- Bruises and sprains
- Cough
- Complaints of the elderly
- Liver and kidney problems,

and many more. In fact, there is hardly an ailment for which there is no simple home remedy easily available.

On the pages ahead, I am going to tell where to find these remedies and how to use them.

Right now they are in your house, unrecognized. They are in your bathroom, your kitchen, your laundry, your broom closet, your driveway, your back yard. Many are free of cost; others low in cost.

They all work.

Frank E., an elderly man, complained of weak eyes that burned and watered constantly. I recommended he drink six ounces of a certain raw vegetable juice, which I will tell you about in Chapter 3. In ten days his eyes were dramatically improved.

I did not invent the remedy. It has been around for years. I thank my grandmother for it, and I'm sure she thanked her grandmother.

John D., a painting contractor, came to me with a chronic stiff neck. It bothered him constantly for years. I gave him what is being called the "Dr. Schneider Neck Exercise." Within a few days his neck improved; in ten days he was discharged pain free.

It is really not *my* exercise. I inherited it. More about it in Chapter 7.

A woman, Mrs. Joy S., came to my office with pain and numbness in her left arm. She could only afford one treatment. I recommended she buy some inexpensive spring-type clothespins and put them on her fingertips five minutes, twice a day. In two weeks she phoned to report the condition ninety percent improved. See Chapter 8 about how this simple remedy works.

THE LABEL "SUPERSTITION" IS BEING CHANGED TO "NATURAL REMEDY"

If you can remember a grandfather or a grandmother, chances are you can just hear that person telling you about sassafras tea. "It's good for what ails you."

Superstition? Not on your life. Thousands of Americans are still drinking sassafras tea today and gaining multiple health benefits from it.

And they are putting on hot packs or cold packs, sipping a glass of sherry ("It's better'n a nurse for old folk"), drinking raw vegetable juices, taking long walks in the fresh air, and doing many of the things that their mothers and fathers stopped doing, but which health care specialists are rediscovering.

Meanwhile, other Americans are discovering that hospitals are full. Doctors are so busy they have to run their offices like a production line. New medicines are being invented faster than doctors can learn about them and use them, yet diseases are increasing even faster.

Man is on the verge of a health care crisis.

It seems every step he takes away from the old ways of natural living and into the modern manufactured, synthesized, plastic life style, the closer he comes to the brink of this health crisis.

I can just see Mother Nature, hands on hips, calling, "Come back. Come back!"

On the pages ahead, I am going to remind you of what your grandparents and their grandparents knew — about remedying ailments — from back to front and from head to toe.

It is great wisdom. Wisdom of the ages. It is both preventive and curative. It is not like modern chemicals where you had best read the fine print describing possible dangerous "side effects." The old-fashioned ways are simple. No "side effects." Just good effects.

These are all natural remedies that have worked, — better for some people than for others. We are all people, but we are different one from the other in subtle ways. On the pages ahead, I have selected those that have worked best in my own experience, or in the experience of people known to me.

Old-fashioned health remedies cover the whole spectrum of human ailments. Although some come in the form of movements, or in the use of hot and cold, or in postures and pressures, many are supplied by nature in the form of edibles.

For instance did you know that:

- Barley water has been used successfully to correct gall and kidney stones and to lower fever, and that cooked barley is said to help prevent tooth decay and loss of hair.
- Oil of eucalyptus, one teaspoonful held in the mouth for ten minutes then swallowed, can head off a cold when you feel one coming on.
- Carob flour, added to the formula of babies, has helped in some cases where they have not been able to keep food down.
- Radishes, eaten raw in salad, have been used to relieve catarrah and excessive mucus.
- Bananas were favored as a soothing food to sufferers of ulcerative colitis.
- Licorice has been used since the days of the ancient Greeks to calm coughs and soothe throat irritations.

THE ORIGINAL MIRACLE WORKER

Nature has endowed every living thing with the intelligence it needs to survive. This intelligence within every person is so vast we cannot intellectually conceive of its magnitude.

Just for starters: Nature strings up a nerve system of communications far more complicated than New York City's telephone system. It stretches muscles and ligaments as if they were guy wires on the George Washington Bridge across the Hudson, each exactly the right length and attached in the right place to do its work. It mixes lime with other minerals extracted from food and engineers bones to withstand with maximum efficiency the stresses and torques which will be brought to bear on them.

Nature completed all this in nine months. If the world's greatest engineers tried to accomplish such a job it might take thousands of years and then get bungled.

Then does the master engineer we call nature walk away from you? No, it stays on the job.

If you have salted herring for lunch, how much water is needed to neutralize the salt? Nature knows and takes care of it.

If you run to catch a bus, how much faster must your heart beat to supply the working parts with their needs? Check your pulse: Nature has already taken care of it.

If you have on four pounds of cotton and polyester clothing and the room temperature is 68° Fahrenheit, how much blood sugar must be burned to maintain your body temperature at 98.6 degrees? Don't try to calculate it. Nature has it figured out and under control.

Our ancestors did not try to upstage nature. Instead, they utilized nature. They let nature do the repairing, recharge the cell batteries, connect the broken circuits, throw out the invader.

Occasionally nature asked for help from them. A chill meant the need for warm blankets. But often the message did not come quite that obviously.

HOW NATURE TOLD THE OLD FOLKS WHAT TO DO

Take the story of Ann Wigmore, a doctor of divinity in Boston, Mass. She remembers two years of nightmare as a child in a remote section of war torn Europe where she grew up. Villagers huddled together in root cellars, waist deep in water as Russians and Germans fought in hand-to-hand battle.

The people emerged from the root cellars at night to gnaw the bark of trees and forage for whatever else they could find to eat. Her grandmother brought back ordinary grass which she chewed for sustenance.

She survived, eventually came to the United States and became a minister. Still sickly, she was reminded of the grass her grandmother used to feed her.

But what kind of grass?

She decided to let nature make the decision. She planted seven different recommended varieties in different pots. When they had grown sufficiently, she let her white kitten into the room. It smelled each wisp of grass. Then it began to chew on the wheatgrass.

Then she tried her neighbor's cocker spaniel. It, too, selected the wheatgrass. Finally, she tried a hungry alley cat. Without any hesitation, it chewed the wheatgrass ravenously.

Today she credits her good health to this natural remedy — as do thousands of others — wheatgrass. Get it in the health food stores. Grow it yourself. Chew on it. Put it in salads. A natural tonic. I recommend wheatgrass to many of my patients.

A cow intuitively moves to the grass in the pasture that is best for her. A poisonous grass, just as green and just as tempting, is ignored. Nature is talking to us constantly.

Ann Wigmore helped perpetuate this particular remedy. She listened to nature.

Chances are most of our grandparents' tried and true recipes came through nature's own signs, signals, and inspiration.

One of nature's messages constantly ignored in the rush of modern times is "take a nap." You feel like it, but for one reason or another you dismiss the urge. Which would you rather have, nervous indigestion or a nap? I recommend the nap.

The old folks used common horse sense. That means they did what comes naturally.

It was natural to grab sixty winks in the middle of the day. You could do it in a rocking chair or a haystack, indoors or out.

In many countries they still have siesta. Everything closes up for a couple of hours.

The nap does not interfere with a night's sleep if taken in the middle of the day. In fact, it can accelerate the falling asleep process come nightfall. You are not overtired, over-stimulated. You are able to get into the mental posture of sleep more readily.

White House doctors have long advised presidents to take time off for a nap in the middle of the day. Some advised the presidents to get into their pajamas, pull the blinds, and turn in just like they do at night. It has been reported that Lyndon Johnson slept as much as three hours during the day and that most Washington legislators manage a fifteen minute nap.

If you have chronic problems such as fatigue, nervousness, a cross temperament, nausea, indigestion, try taking a nap as a regular mid-day procedure. When we sleep we give nature a chance to do its normalizing, harmonizing, and balancing work, without the interference of our conscious mind. Most of us, through tension, harbor emotions, thoughts, and attitudes that are negative, unharmonious, and unbalancing. Just a few minutes of sleep permits the body to normalize and adjust itself.

Sleep is therapeutic. We know that. They knew it in times gone by, too, but they gave it more of a chance. Today we are too busy. It's only when the body begins to complain that, maybe, we begin to pay more attention to the benefits of sleep.

Tom and Mary S. were having a problem with their marriage. When the husband came home from a hard day's work, the wife took out all her troubles on him, not realizing it. They both came to me for a nerve tonic. I prescribed a nap.

He figured a way to catch a few winks in the office after lunch. She did the same thing at home. In three days they were acting like they were on their second honeymoon.

Even if you don't have a complaint, I prescribe a nap — daily.

You are going to be surprised at the common products, materials, and actions that constitute genuine, effective remedies. Take garlic. It is in every kitchen. It could also be in your medicine chest, it is that powerful a remedy.

George B., 13, was weak. He had been through a number of tests without any clues. I gave him garlic. The garlic ended a case of worms. He was his young, energetic self again.

I have recommended garlic for a number of young teenagers, whom I suspected might have intestinal worms, and in a majority of cases the mothers have told me of finding worms that were expelled in the stools. The easiest way of using garlic for a suspected worm case is to obtain the garlic capsules sold in your health food stores.

Another effective use of garlic which I have recommended so many times is in the cases of hypertensive high blood pressure. This may not be a complete control, but it is helpful used along with other measures to help control high blood pressure. Like anything else, some people respond better than others to garlic for hypertension. Either take garlic in capsule form or use liberally in two or three food items daily.

Today, scientists are showing a new respect for old-fashioned remedies. They are examining the medical folklore of the American Indian, exploring African witch doctor healing methods and even the South Seas for secrets of the ancient Kahunas. However, one mistake keeps being made over and over again.

THE ONE INGREDIENT THAT ONLY NATURE HAS

The scientists take a good natural cure back into the laboratory, analyze its chemical composition, then synthesize the substance from the same chemicals.

When the synthetic substance doesn't work as well, they wonder why.

I'll tell you why. Nature has not told them about a secret ingredient – *organic life force.* You cannot see organic life force under a microscope. Nor can you synthesize it.

Need iron? Munching on iron filings will not do a bit of good. It is missing organic life force.

Now, if you put the iron into soil in which leafy vegetables are growing, and you eat the vegetables, you receive the iron in a form that your body uses and thrives on.

Old fashioned remedies often work best because they are natural remedies – not synthetic imitations – *natural* remedies, brimming with a secret ingredient that carries within it the very force we call life.

No old-fashioned remedies will die with me. I hope to perpetuate them, not only in my practice, but through my patients who will be somebody's grandparents some day – and through this book. I use many of these on myself and in my growing practice, – rubs, movements, poultices, foods.

There is a movement, a stretching I have recommended more than any other. I also use it myself regularly to tone and stretch the back muscles with the lower back muscles particularly involved. It goes like this: Lying on the back, draw the knees (bent) up to the abdomen. Clasp the hands over the shins (if impossible, over the knees), pulling the legs as closely as possible to the abdomen. Slacken the grip, then tighten again, repeating until the lower back feels the stretch (pull).

Just plain ordinary food used to be more healthful in the old days than today. Chemical pesticides and chemical fertilizers add nothing to food value. Good old horse and sheep manure made the soil rich. Vegetables in Europe today, where they still care for the soil in nature's way, have many times the taste and nutritional value of our vegetables.

One of my patients carried on a family tradition, despite new sprays available. He used a concoction of red pepper and garlic on his cherry trees. They were right across the road from mine. I did not use sprays either. But I can tell you his were mighty fine cherries — and twice the yield of mine.

There. I've saved that idea from being lost to posterity.

Country folk still see all sorts of signs in nature. Bees hovering over their hives in a restless and disturbed manner means that a downpour is on the way. An old formula for telling the temperature still works where there are crickets — count the number of chirps per fifteen seconds and add forty.

Robins sing energetically before rain. Seagulls sense an approaching storm, flying inland to safer terrain. Spiders, expecting rain, strengthen their webs.

You don't have to worry about the birds or the bees forgetting nature's secrets. It's man that needs to be reminded.

COMMON REMEDIES THAT WILL GO ON FOREVER

Nobody is going to forget that old saying, "An apple a day keeps the doctor away." But fewer and fewer people are doing anything about it.

Of course, now that doctors don't make house calls, we have to change that to "An apple a day keeps you away from the doctor."

It is still true — in spirit. Apples are still good for you. But chances are they are not all as good for you as they used to be.

First of all, there's all that chemical spray. Even if you wash the apple you are still eating some of the chemical poisons. Over the long run, that can bring you to the doctor.

Second, you may lose the benefit through cooking. Apples are often boiled with sugar, bottled, and canned, and all you've got is applesauce. The good is out and a new threat to health put in.

You don't ever get the old favorite kinds of apples any more. Remember the Winesaps, Roman Beauties, Baldwins and Newtons? You seldom see those around, and they were the highest in vitamin C. They were the tart tasting kind. Today, people go for the blander delicious varieties which have less than a quarter of the amount of vitamin C.

Grandma knew the difference. She knew what "good" meant. She knew it meant not just good to your tastebuds, but good to all of you. Start thinking about crisp, tart apples because in a few pages I am going to be telling you all the good things they can do for you.

Grandma knew a lot of things that Mother never learned. The skillful housewife a hundred years ago made bread and ground the meat herself. She made soap, beer, ink, salves, tinctures, bandages. She knew how to milk a cow, churn butter, scrub clothes. She treated ringworm and measles in her family, while at the same time in the farmyard she treated bloat in cattle and gapes in chickens.

Grandma knew the value of roots, barks, herbs, flowers, seeds, leaves, and gums. And if she did not know, she could ask her grandma or grandpa.

People in the country survived harsh and rugged conditions largely because they had nature's remedies close at hand.

In the old-time cities, it was a different story. Maybe living conditions were more comfortable and protected than in the country, but this was often at the sacrifice of adequate sanitation.

Hospitals were avoided like the plague. And just as unsuccessfully. There, squalor prevailed and epidemics broke out, with typhus and typhoid fever taking the lives of half the patients at such hospitals as New York's Bellevue in the mid-1880's.

So we don't look back at those times necessarily as the good old days. But if we are able to sift the good from the bad, we can make an attempt to preserve the best of the good.

For instance, examine tranquilizers. The pills being popped in the millions today are assaults on the body that leave some patients progressively more damaged by them. For centuries before these pills were made, people relied on a natural tranquilizer — wine.

John G. came to see me. He was 64, facing retirement. It was causing him uneasiness. He became fidgety, irritable. Did I have a pill to calm his nerves?

I had something better, I told him — a glass of wine every afternoon. It proved to be "just what the doctor ordered" in calming John.

Wine is one of the oldest and safest medicines in the world. I'll be saying a good deal about the juice of grapes later, but as a tranquilizer, wine is nature's prescription. Nurses in some homes for the aged go around administering pills to keep everybody calm. You'd think you were in a living cemetery. If they would let the old folks sip a glass of wine once or twice during the day, it would be a healthier and happier atmosphere.

Can the tranquilizing pills prevent infectious diseases, like the natural antibiotics in wine can? Or protect against anemia? Or provide ready energy? Wine does this. Wine will always be with us. Its ancient medicinal uses, as stated in the Bible, may be forgotten, but remembered or not, the glass of wine performs its natural "therapy."

Feel on edge? Instead of taking a tranquilizer, try a few sips of wine. Make it red wine. You will feel good, calm, yet not sedated.

The simple things in life often turn out to be the best. Who has not been tortured at one time or another by a stuffed-up nose? It is a bothersome symptom that is an inevitable part of the common cold syndrome. Some people go through periods of sinus problems, giving them a chronic breathing difficulty. Many people who use the modern sprays and drops find that temporary relief is paid for by even tighter blocking later.

Take the case of Grandma W., now in her 80's. For twenty years she could not breathe through the left side of her nose, and headaches troubled her for years. I recommended the normal saline solution for her. You heard me right. Salt.

The next time Grandma W. came to my office she was jubilant as a young girl. "Look Doc." She used her finger and closed the right side of her nose showing me she could breathe through the previously closed left side. Her headaches and the tight, stuffy feeling she had in her nose and head were gone. She told me that at first it was very difficult to get the solution back into her nose. The next time she used the solution, she expelled a large, dark glob of mucus. From that time on her condition greatly improved.

This salt water remedy will go on forever. Try it next time you have this problem. Use a shallow bowl. Sniffle it well up into your nose. You will have quick relief. (Complete detail in later chapter)

The rubs, juices, and compresses that I am going to tell you about in the chapters ahead will also go on forever. Take a simple thing, like an ice pack.

In order to have ice all year round, our forefathers had to go out in the late winter and cut blocks of ice from a frozen lake. Then they would haul these blocks to an ice house where they would be stored, covered with sawdust.

These days ice for ice packs comes a lot easier, so there is every reason in the world to know when an ice pack can relieve a bothersome condition.

Frances A. had suffered with migraine headaches for fifteen years. I had treated her several times. Sometimes the standard chiropractic treatment would be effective, and sometimes it would not. Now she was on the phone asking for another treatment.

A holiday weekend was approaching, and I had made plans to be out of town, so I could not treat her in person. She asked if there was anything I could recommend to give her relief until I returned to my office. I suggested a remedy that I had successfully used previously with other migraine patients. I explained to her that I felt the blood was not circulating or draining properly from the brain. I suggested she fill a water bag with ice water. I told her to put the soles of her feet on the water bag and cover herself with a light blanket. She was to lie down in this position for thirty minutes to one hour.

Later, just as I was about to leave, Frances A. phoned to report that her headache was gone. "This has worked better than anything," she said.

This was some time ago. Recently the Menninger Clinic here in Topeka, Kansas, where I live, reported on some work they were doing with biofeedback equipment to help migraine sufferers. The patient would cause his hands to become hot merely thinking them to be hot. This would activate the circulation system to send more blood to the hands.

More blood in the hands relieved the headache, apparently due to too much blood being in the head. They say headaches are traceable to too much pressure or tension. So the blood goes to where the problem is. The wisdom of this old cold pack remedy is more appreciated in the light of modern science.

The specific remedies recommended for specific ailments should not be interpreted as a cure for their specific conditions, but only as an aid in conjunction with other therapies, including cause removal, to stimulate, help heal, or cleanse a certain portion of the body that is not functioning up to normal. The general idea is to use these remedies or recommendations to balance out all systems of the body. The body functions as one unit and can not be separated, dissected, or torn apart to treat one system of the body at a time, forgetting about all of the other systems.

We may not readily understand why stretching this or pressing that works, either. Or why beet juice will help you in one way and carrot juice in another. But most of us don't understand how electricity works, but we use it anyhow.

Every time I hear a nutritionist mention how a certain food is high in this mineral or that vitamin, I nod my head knowingly. That's why the old timers used it as a remedy. I like to trust nature as Grandma did.

And Grandma sure knew what she was doing.

2

HOW YOU CAN MAKE THE SUPERMARKET YOUR GOLD MINE FOR HEALTH

Do you know what a "love apple" is?

Guess again. It's a tomato — the fruit that we eat as a vegetable. It is a native of South America, imported to the United States centuries ago, but not taken seriously until our grandparents' generation.

In fact, until then, white Americans would not eat a tomato for love or money. They called it the "love apple" because it was believed to be poisonous to everybody except people in love. Indians, a lot closer to nature, recognized the good in tomatoes. Soon Indians were raising them and people began to call tomatoes "Indian apples." That made our grandfolks think twice. If tomatoes were considered good by the Indians, they must be worth eating.

Tomatoes are indeed worth eating. These and other foods rank high on the list of nature's remedies that will always be used because they work best.

Most of these remedy foods are in your supermarket, not your pharmacy. They are not labeled as "good for arthritis" or "natural laxative" or "heart balm." They are labeled tomatoes, grapes, etc. In this chapter I hope I make you so conscious of these special fruits and vegetables that whenever you go by them, you will see the word "remedy" light up on them.

Nature's remedies are also preventive. You don't have to be suffering from a liver disease in order for certain meats plus the juice of grapes to be good for you. Just eating these foods can lessen your chances for being susceptible to the unwanted condition.

So the purpose of this chapter in highlighting certain supermarket foods is to prevent as well as to relieve symptoms. I'll tell you what foods to favor with your food budget in order to keep your level of resistance to disease high.

Let's describe the foods that I am now going to recommend to you as the kinds of foods that can keep the "miseries" away from your door; that decrease the likelihood of your catching cold, grippe, or flu; and that cut down on your visits to the doctor for soreness, aches, pains, nerves and other complaints. These are the foods that will keep you young and spry, full of nature's zeal, zest, and zip.

FRUITS AND VEGETABLES THAT YOU SHOULD GET TO KNOW BETTER

Put these high on your shopping list:

Spinach	Cabbage
Turnip greens	Dandelion greens
Mustard greens	Taro tops
Escarole	Broccoli
Kale	Collard

These leafy green vegetables are brimming with vitamins and minerals that your body cells hunger for — like calcium, iron, potassium, vitamins A, B, C, E, and K.

Calcium helps build bones, teeth, and nails. Good for the nerves, too. Got muscle cramps, menstrual pains? You may need calcium — available from these leafy greens.

Iron helps the blood to do its job of carrying oxygen to cells everywhere. Lack of iron results in anemia, listlessness, lack of mental alertness.

Potassium is a muscle mineral, so it is important to such muscle functions as heart action and bowel evacuation.

With lots of vitamin A your new body cells grow vigorously, so you show a high resistance to infections and an increase in longevity.

With lots of vitamin B digestion is good and nerves are stable. You have a healthy appetite.

With lots of vitamin C, the mucous tissue is healthier, so are the teeth and gums, and your body makes bone marrow and hormones like it should.

With lots of vitamin E, your muscles are regenerated and show good tone.

With lots of vitamin K, your blood coagulates normally and prevents excessive bleeding or hemorrhaging.

With lots of spinacn and other leafy vegetables you get these important minerals and vitamins.

In the fruit department, you know the kind I'm going to point to first — and generations of old folk are looking over my shoulder, nodding their head in agreement.

"Pick the tart apple, not the Delicious variety," they are urging.

Mrs. S. complained of a tired, rundown feeling she'd had for several months. She appeared to have been taking enough vitamin foods, but after questioning her about her diet, I found she was eating far too many bread products and not enough fruits and vegetables. She also complained of constipation. She said she felt well until the middle of the morning and then tired for the remainder of the day.

I asked her to enjoy a nice, big, fresh raw apple for breakfast and to eat it instead of her morning breakfast roll. A week later she returned to my office. She raved about having a wonderful, more energetic feeling throughout the entire day. Most of her constipation problem had disappeared, thanks to the bulk in her diet from eating the raw apples.

More about what the curative powers of the apple can do for you later.

THE OLD WIVES' TALE THAT HAS NOW BEEN PROVEN TRUE

Bulk is important to our diet. What we mean by bulk is fiber. This is largely removed from the prepared foods we find in the supermarket. In former times, it was never a problem. People got plenty of bulk in whole grains, fruits, and vegetables.

Today whole grains are the exception, depleted grains are the rule. Some doctors think that lack of bulk is the reason for cancer of the colon and of the rectum, now becoming second only to lung cancer as the leading cause of death due to malignancy.

A study made of American blacks showed that their ancestors in African villages hardly experienced colonic cancer. Then the sons and daughters who came to America, who still tried to hold to the same diet, got the disease about half as frequently as American whites. Today's blacks, with the diet now largely the same as whites, get the disease on a par with today's whites.

Many health care specialists still belittle the importance of roughage. They think it is an old wives' tale. I say all the more reason to perk up our ears if the old wives believed it.

Here's the way the researchers explain it. Refined diets take longer to be eliminated. Longer transit time in the bowels permit bacteria-produced cancer-producing agents more contact with the bowel linings.

I recommend that you eat some roughage food daily. It cleanses your system.

Get your roughage from the following supermarket foods:

Fruits	*Vegetables*	*Grains*
Apples	Beets	Corn
Berries	Cabbage	Whole wheat bread
Pears	Cauliflower	Whole wheat cereal
	Brussels Sprouts	Bran cereal
	Tomatoes	
	Eggplant	
	Broccoli	
	Summer squash	

Before you leave the vegetable department, take a good look at the carrots and beets. They are old friends. I'll tell their health secrets later.

HERBS FOR BETTER HEALTH AND COOKERY

Herbs used to be the only medicine available. And people survived on them when needed.

I will be referring to certain herbs as specific remedies in the chapters ahead, but right now I want to turn the spotlight on the

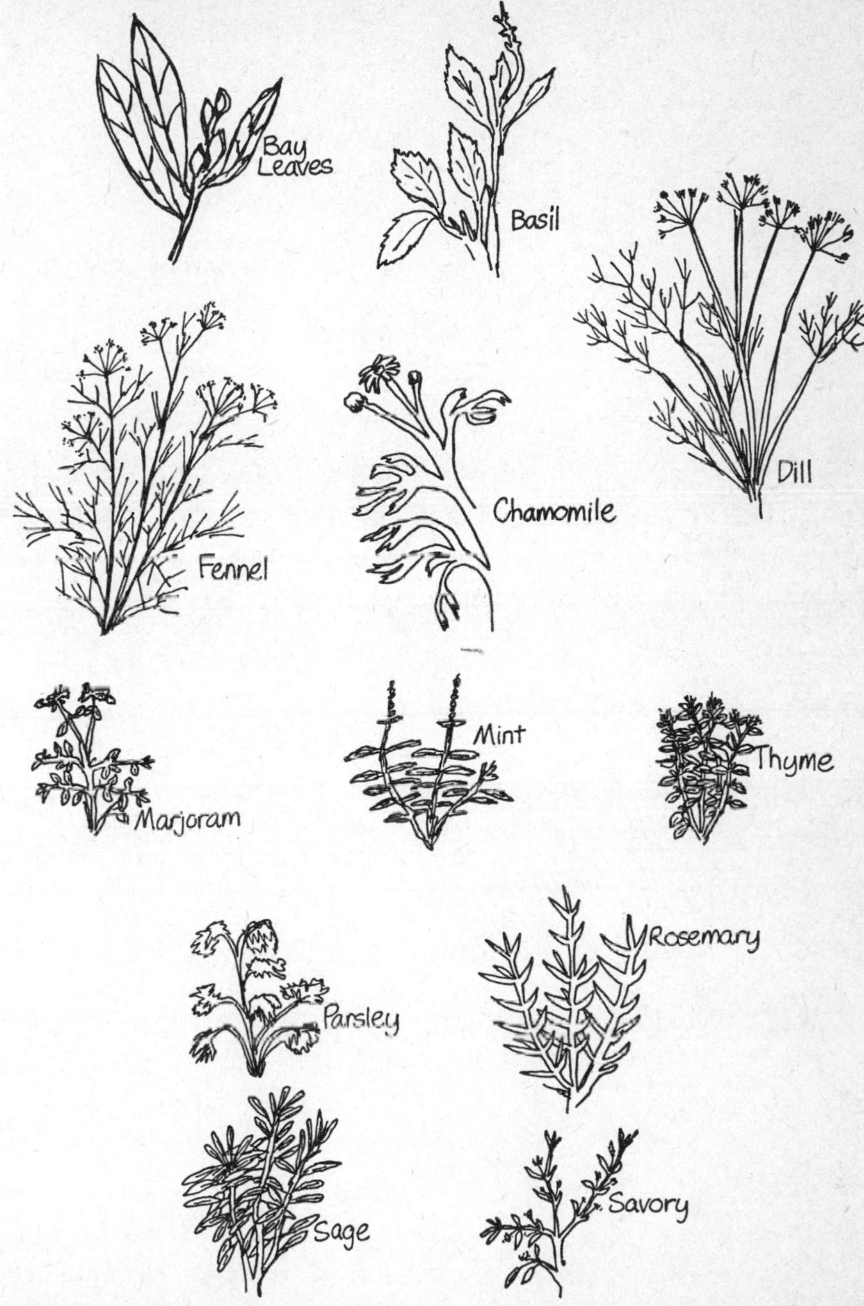
Bay Leaves
Basil
Dill
Fennel
Chamomile
Marjoram
Mint
Thyme
Rosemary
Parsley
Sage
Savory

Figure 2-1

kinds of herbs that the old timers kept in stock to flavor their food and brew tea — knowing that even dried and bottled they still bring to your body the vitality that nature has stored in them.

When you pass the herb and spice counter, you might like to pick up some of these herbs and get to know them better. *Figure 2-1* shows twelve reliable remedies:

Basil —	often used in cooking meat and fish. Was considered an antiseptic and frequently used as *sedative, laxative, expectorant, and for reducing temperatures.*
Bay Leaves —	Aunt Mathilda kept bay leaves around for many complaints, especially to *apply on rheumatic joints.* In the kitchen she used bay leaves for marinading and preserving.
Chamomile —	Still used in Europe as a tea, *helpful to digestion* after a heavy meal.
Dill —	Another *good-for-digestion* herb, but also used as a flavoring. Grandma used to try to get the old man to chew dill seeds to kill the smell of tobacco.
Fennel —	An old favorite to flavor the trout that the men folk brought home, it can also be used *to soothe inflammation of the eyes.*
Marjoram —	Tastes like meat loaf because that's where it was usually hidden. *Peps up a dull appetite* and has antiseptic qualities. Said to have been a favorite for the typical snakebite patent medicines.
Mint —	Used as a tea, a good bracer, as well as a *stomach settler.* A favorite in Colonial kitchens, especially for its help to digestion.
Parsley —	A vitamin-rich herb (A, B, and C). *Helps decrease stomach gas* and said to help combat rheumatic pain.
Rosemary —	When not used as a flavoring for beef casseroles and sauces, it is used therapeutically for digestion and *stimulating blood circulation* to parts where it is applied externally.
Sage —	For centuries a life giving tea and *general health tonic* throughout most of the world.

Savory — Used to flavor grandma's baked beans because it helped *combat flatulence* that beans are notorious for.

Thyme — A favorite in the kitchen for making crab apple jelly, thyme was also found in the linen and lace drawers as a scented sachet and in the sick room as a gargle and *disinfectant.*

Many of the above herbs have more than one health use. One might work better for a particular person than it does for another person with the same problem. Take parsley.

Many patients who have complained of tiredness between meals are delighted that I advised them about parsley. I recommended that they chew a few sprigs of parsley with their meal, as parsley is an energy food. Parsley is one of the highest proteins, if not the highest in the vegetable kingdom. It is also high in other nutrients.

Mrs. Alice H. should not have been constantly fatigued. In her early forties, happily married and the mother of two fine children, she was in the prime of life. In response to her complaint, I recommended she decorate every meal with parsley, then eat the decoration. Within two weeks she was "a new woman."

Another recommendation in the use of parsley is for its deodorizing effect. For those who have extremely profuse body and/or foot odors, it is excellent to neutralize them. Parsley is much safer than some of the anti-perspirants on the market.

The secret deodorizing ingredient of parsley is its chlorophyl.

I was told by a professional chef that the reason for parsley garnishing a favorite steak is not only for the appearance or plate dressing, but for the diner to chew after he has eaten the steak, reducing the halitosis which most people have after eating meat.

LOOK ON THE SALAD DRESSING SHELVES FOR THIS HEALTH-GIVING FOOD

Much has been written about this old country favorite, so I won't say too much about it, except that tucked away on the supermarket shelves among all sorts of salad dressings is — apple cider vinegar. Pressed for specific cures that apple cider may be good for, the country store proprietor would usually just say, "It's good for what ails you."

I mentioned several remedial uses for apple cider vinegar in the previous chapter. Here is another.

I have used apple cider vinegar as a kidney stimulator. If a sluggish kidney condition has been plaguing you, perhaps this kidney remedy will help. It sure can't hurt you.

The vinegar supplies many of the essential elements so necessary for good kidney function and body chemistry. One of the main reasons that vinegar is beneficial is because it supplies needed potassium to the system. Potassium is often lacking to such a large degree that it causes a poor flushing of the kidney. The body can also be low in acid. The vinegar supplies a natural acid.

Over my years in practice I have had both young and elderly patients complain of scanty urination. Their liquid intake would be normal. There would be very little evidence of tissue fluid (edema). Their stools would not be hard or compacted. They had, in fact, rather normal bowel movements. But there did not seem to be a normal volume of urine excreted in a 24-hour period. The best remedy I have found for this condition is to mix one teaspoon of apple cider vinegar for every 50 pounds of body weight with a glass of water and consume with each meal. In most cases, I have the patient use this for two days, and then let the kidneys rest for four days.

Mr. A., age 65, was probably a classic example. He would urinate three or four times per day very scantily. After using apple cider vinegar for 24 hours, he urinated ten times the first day. He continued using this preparation for one week after which he told me he then was urinating six to eight times a day with a lot more volume than being excreted each time before. He felt much better.

SPICES AS A SUPERMARKET HEALTH SOURCE

Near the herbs in most markets, and maybe intermingled with them, are spices. Actually, the two are pretty mixed up in people's minds, too. Technically speaking spices are bark, roots, leaves, stems, buds, seeds, and fruits of aromatic plants, many of which grow in the tropics, while herbs are just the leaves of plants, most of which grow in temperate zones, and are also usually aromatic in character.

Spices were too valuable in the old days to be in everybody's kitchen. They came by boat from India and the Orient, usually, and were considered "treasure." Ships with spice were prime targets for piracy.

The aromatic character of a spice is nature's way of saying "look at me — I'm bursting with goodness for you." If the exotic fragrance of distant lands does not greet your sense of taste or smell when you open a spice container, chances are it is stale and needs replacing.

Seeds contain the germ of life. Seeds planted centuries later still grow. I think spices that are seeds are certainly good spices to have around. On your supermarket shelf you'll see:

Anise Seed —	It has a licorice flavor and is used for cookies and on coffee cake and sweet rolls.
Caraway Seed —	Used in sauerkraut and in making rye bread.
Cardamon Seed —	Used also in baking, and as a flavoring in grape jelly.
Cumin Seed —	A real old spice used in chili and curry powders. On its own, good in soups.
Mustard Seed —	Also blended with other spices, as in prepared mustard. On its own — chopped meat, salad, fish.
Poppy Seed —	Nearly one million of these tiny seeds to the pound. Aunt Martha used them as a topping for that fresh bread she baked, all rolls, and cookies.
Sesame Seed —	Small and honey colored, these seeds are one of the main ingredients of the candy halvah. Popularly used in baking.

Two excellent seeds are seldom found in supermarkets or grocery stores, but are usually available in health food stores. These are sunflower seeds and pumpkin seeds.

Sunflower seeds are quite popular in the Soviet Union where they are munched right from the pocket throughout the day — and at the motion picture shows like we munch on popcorn. What a difference in nutritional value! Life-giving seeds versus life-sapping butterfat.

Pumpkin seeds are becoming almost as popular in the United States. With the hard outer shells removed (de-shelled), they are an excellent source of vitamins, minerals, proteins, and trace elements. I have recommended pumpkin seeds (de-shelled) for intestinal worms with very good results in a number of cases of children whom I have treated over the years.

I remember a particular case many years ago of Tommy F., — a youngster who was underweight and tired and run-down most of the time. I suspected he had intestinal worms. I had Tommy's parents obtain pumpkin seeds, allowing him to eat as many de-shelled seeds daily as he cared for. Within a few weeks Tommy had attained a normal weight for his age and had more strength and energy. Although the parents did not report finding worms expelled in his stools, he had regained more health after using the pumpkin seeds.

Pumpkin seeds have a reputation for preventing prostate trouble in men. I have not had any professional experience with pumpkin seeds in these cases, but any man faced with prostate trouble might try pumpkin seeds. They won't hurt. In fact, their zinc content can be just what your prostate needs.

We are talking about spices now, not just seeds, so I want to take a moment to tell you about one spice on your supermarket shelves that has a special use.

A COMMON SPICE WITH AN UNUSUAL BENEFIT

The spice is cloves. In cooking it is used in pork and ham roasts, pickled fruits, and spiced syrups. Another use has been handed down from person to person through the years — it helps you to cut down on smoking.

A patient, Margaret C., told me that years before her father had been an extremely heavy smoker. He had tried various ways to break the habit but to no avail. Then he heard about cloves. He used them and quit smoking entirely.

I was quite interested in Margaret's story, so I tried this remedy myself. Although I did not quit smoking entirely, it did help reduce the number of cigarettes I smoked per day. I have suggested this remedy to a number of patients and have found it to give equally good results. This inexpensive therapy certainly is worth trying to overcome an expensive habit.

Here is how it works:

The nicotine taste that is left in the mouth after smoking is one of the causes for reaching for another cigarette, pipe, or cigar. Cloves, in my opinion, have a more or less neutralizing effect on this taste.

The best type of cloves to keep well moistened in the mouth is the type which can be purchased at the spice counter in the grocery store.

Take one small branch, and after having it in the mouth for two hours, discard and use another fresh clove branch.

This inexpensive method is definitely worth a try if you want to lessen or break the habit of smoking.

HOW TO GET IN YOUR OWN WAY IN THE SUPERMARKET

Outdoor and sheltered booths where farmers could offer their wares used to be an American way of life. Now, however, there are middlemen, using new ways of food processing and packaging. Life-containing goodness is extracted, and in its place go chemical preservatives. Now there is no need to send these foods directly from farm to market. The route is farm to factory to warehouse to railroad or freighter to another warehouse to the supermarket.

There the packages, cans, and jars can stand for up to months and not spoil. Even bread, with the wheat germ out and freshness preserving chemicals in, can be kept for days and still feel soft to the buyer's touch. Not a worm or insect would go near this bread, as it contains no live nourishment.

Refined sugar is another example. When sugar is refined, the life energy comes out in the molasses. At one time the dumping of molasses in Cuba became a public health hazard because of its attracting bugs and gnats, causing them to breed and multiply on these rich nutrients — which had been removed!

Supermarkets still have the original farm-to-market type of food. Get to recognize which areas have "alive" foods and which "dead" foods. Fresh fruits and vegetables are your best bet. Then the dairy items, with a nod to natural cheeses versus processed cheese. Choose fresh and unprocessed meat, poultry, and fish, wherever possible. Avoid smoked varieties — smoking may enhance the flavor and shelf-life but it does nothing for *you*. Hot dogs with nitrates and nitrites and other chemicals (read the labels) are not worthy of their popularity. Sausages and wursts are usually also chemically treated.

These chemicals get in the way of your own life-support systems. Buy the unchemicalized foods.

You are better off doing your own cooking than buying frozen vegetables, for instance, which need to be only partially cooked. And you are better off buying fresh foods and doing the cooking yourself than buying canned foods.

Canning may involve pre-cooking and preservatives, and the water and heat dissolves and injures many vitamins and minerals. Canning also involves adding sugar — as with most canned fruits. Sugar is the cause of many of our health problems today — from tooth decay to arthritis including the underlying cause of many critical disorders, obesity.

Frozen and canned foods are convenience foods. It is good to have some around for that occasional quick meal. And an *occasional* processed food never hurt anybody. It's making processed foods your life style that can take its toll.

So are the cake mixes, pastries, and other boxed foods a convenience. But don't let yourself be hypnotized by the "instant" promise of puddings made from mixes.

You are better off to ignore the hard sell in big print and instead read the truth about what is in the package in fine print.

Fill those shopping carts with melons, apples, grapes, and berries. Don't skimp on fresh fruits. Automatically reach for *fresh* beets, celery, lettuce, greens of all types, squash, carrots, and other fresh vegetables. Even shell the peas yourself rather than buy canned or frozen peas, if fresh peas are available. That's what your mother did. And her mother.

Look for low fat, natural cheeses. Sun dried (non-sulphured) raisins, figs, dates, and apricots are great nutritional foods. Try molasses, real maple syrup, and honey instead of white sugar. Brown sugar is really refined sugar with some of the molasses put back in. That's better than white. Favor the more natural brown rice over white rice, whole-wheat bread over white.

Read the labels. Look for nature's goodness. Get the message?

LIFE-GIVING FRUIT JUICES IN THE MARKETPLACE

One good development in the mass marketing of food has come with the bottled juices. In the old days, a farmer with a press was the most popular man around come apple picking time. The apples went into the press and out came apple cider. You could drink it on the spot or take it home in jugs for later. And if it was much later — hard apple cider or even applejack.

Many fruit juices are now available in their natural state — no sugar or preservatives added. These are the remedies. Get them in bottles in preference to cans.

Grape juice is a real old favorite as a natural remedy. I'll be giving you specific ways that grape juice helps you.

So is apple juice. You can now buy brands of apple juice that claim to be made from organically grown apples. This is a term used and often abused. If used properly, it means that no chemicals are placed in the soil as fertilizer, only naturally composed fertilizer is used, and that no sprays are used on the tree or fruit.

When apples were first recognized to be an important natural remedy, that is the way they grew — organically. Nature's way. If you can buy juice of organically grown apples you are buying one of nature's original remedies. Man-made changes have not been exactly therapeutic. Some brands also are made unfiltered. They are cloudier than filtered type. I believe some of the good may be lost in the filtering.

So my sense of priority in apple juice is to buy the organic and the unfiltered, one or the other or both. But if neither is available, don't pass up other kinds of apple juice. They contain much of nature's healing magic, too.

Citric juices are at their best when freshly squeezed from the fruit. You may prefer the convenience of these juices in cans and bottles, but you surely pay for it in lower taste and vitamin content. Frozen orange and grapefruit juice is excellent. But be sure to read the label and make sure you are getting pure juice, without flavoring, color, or sugar added.

A variety of juices is available in bottles now. I have seen pear juice, cranberry juice, even pomegranate juice.

Here is the order of health priority: freshly squeezed juice (by you), frozen juice, bottled juice, canned juice.

Walk slowly when you reach these juices in the supermarket. They are reaching out to you.

HOW TO KEEP THE NUTRITION IN FOODS UNTIL EATEN

Grandma would say, "You look run down."

Grandpa would say, "You've got thin blood."

Chances are they were both talking about the same ailment — anemia. In those days, anybody with that pale look or a general under par feeling was suspected of having this disease, which is a type of malnutrition.

Anemia can come from a diet of foods which are deficient in some way. Or, it can come from foods that were rich in nutrients — before cooking — but are now deficient because of cooking.

You can arrive home from the supermarket laden with life-giving food and still serve yourself and your family an anemia-producing fare.

Albert B.'s case is an example of this. Although only in his forties, he complained of a weak, rundown, tired feeling "most of the time." Albert's main problem was that everything had to be cooked, and cooked well at that to satisfy his taste. He told me that he did not care for any food that was raw.

I explained to him that, by cooking food, a lot of the enzymes are sometimes destroyed, and enzymes are important for digestion and assimilation of the nutrition present in our food.

I suggested that Albert eat raw celery, radishes, lettuce — in fact, to have a nice fresh vegetable salad with each meal. He promised to do so. In thirty days he returned to my office and told me how much energy he now had. His complexion looked more alive. He said that by eating the salads he ate less of the canned foods. His elimination had greatly improved. He felt better, had more energy, and looked years younger.

Look for ways to retain the goodness of the food you bring home from the supermarket. Here are some ways borrowed from our Colonial forbears:

- Keep fresh fruit and vegetables cool.
- Do not slice or cut up until needed.

- Use a minimum of water when cooking.
- Low temperature methods of cooking (like baking) are preferred over high (like frying).
- Cook as little as possible.
- Eat some raw food every day.

The vastness of the variety offered in modern supermarkets is the key to avoiding the most common type of general anemia. Your daily menus should reflect this balanced variety.

Every day should include a dairy product; meat, poultry or fish; a cereal, whole grain if possible; green and yellow vegetables; and fruit.

Keep each of these foods as close to the way nature provides them as your taste permits.

Some excellent roots and herbs are not in your supermarket. Take ginseng.

Ginseng root, prized by the Chinese, is being rediscovered by Americans. Ginseng is found growing wild in the Applachian Mountains and as far west as Kentucky and Eastern Tennessee. It is cultivated in the northern Mid-West — Wisconsin especially. It cost several dollars an ounce.

What does ginseng do for you? In China the men use it as an aphrodisiac, making old men behave like young men again. Methinks that is probably what has made ginseng suddenly become popular in the United States now, too.

But Chinese medical doctors prescribe it as a general tonic, especially for old age complaints and weakness. So powerful is it, the Chinese say, that when a man is faced with death and he needs a few more days to straighten out his affairs, a cup of ginseng tea will do it.

The charisma of ginseng blurs its specific remedial uses, but I place these in areas of exhaustion, impotence, lack of appetite, rheumatic aches and pains, and general down-in-the-mouth feelings.

What was that you said? Yes, it's good for women, too. Check your health food store. I prefer the American or Canadian ginseng to the Korean-grown. *(Figure 2-2)*

Here is how to use ginseng. Wash a small or medium size root.

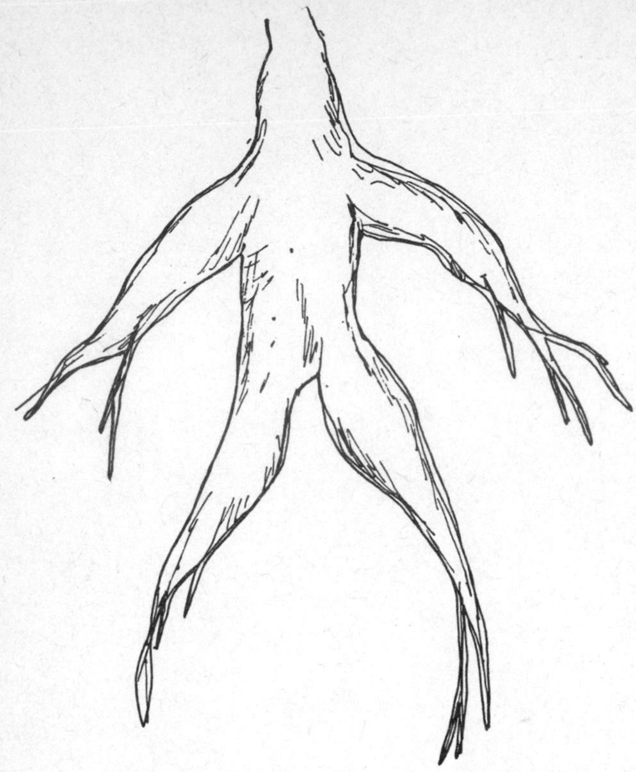

Figure 2-2

Ginseng Root

Put it in a pot of water — about four cups. And simmer for at least an hour. Your ginseng tea is ready. Drink two or three cups a day until you are feeling your young self again.

Russell H. kept ginseng tea going in his store all the time. He could afford to — he grew it. At the age of 70, he looked 50, and apparently felt even younger. He was a robust, active man and he attributed his youthful energy to ginseng.

The older generation had ways of treating ailments that were unique. Some old-fashioned remedies were simply unbelievable. But they worked. And they still work. For instance, without food or medicine:

You can stimulate a vital organ
You can get rid of back pains

You can relieve constipation

You can improve your every day energy

You can accomplish without cost, and for yourself, scores of health improvements.

Here we go.

3

SPECIAL FOODS THAT EXERT AMAZING CURATIVE POWER OVER SUPPOSEDLY INCURABLE CONDITIONS

Farmers used to bring home wild asparagus which they found growing among meadow grasses, if they happened to think about it.

But if a member of the family had an attack of kidney pains or rheumatism, wild asparagus was one of the first things they thought about.

Asparagus in its cultivated form today is just as good a remedy. It helps arthritics, too.

The juice of raw asparagus is the most concentrated way you can take this remedy. Otherwise, cook it normally, stalks first, then the tops down in the water.

Why does asparagus help with kidney pains, rheumatic pain and arthritic pain? The pioneers did not ask why. If they ate something that helped with a problem, they told somebody else about it. The word spread, and was handed down from grandmother to mother.

Along came chemical laboratories. They analyzed asparagus and other old-fashioned remedies and shook their heads. "This food contains nothing special that other foods don't have in equal concentration and abundance."

But the old folks trusted nature's chemical laboratories — their own bodies. Your body is just as trustworthy.

Have you ever noticed how just a couple of hours after eating asparagus, you can smell it when you urinate? What other vegetable acts this way?

Some authorities now report that the juice of asparagus helps to break up oxalic acid crystals in the kidneys as well as elsewhere in the muscles of the body. This would certainly explain how it works as a remedy but not why it works.

I may occasionally tell you what good we know to be in a food remedy, but I am not going to try to explain why special food remedies work. We should be grateful to our great-aunts and great-uncles for passing the word along. Accept the "what" and forget the "why"; nature does not always share her secrets.

A VEGETABLE JUICE THAT RELIEVES STIFF JOINTS

Severe arthritic stiffness may be helped by this simple therapy of drinking six ounces of celery juice daily. This food, thanks to its high sodium content, relieves much of the pain and discomfort of stiff joints. What it may be doing is to help to break down the calcium deposits which have formed and which cause the affliction.

Besides the sodium, celery also contains potassium, calcium, chlorine, phosphorus, sulfur, magnesium, and iron — plus vitamins A, B, C, and E. In my opinion, the reason for celery being beneficial in arthritic conditions is that it supplies some of the minerals which a lack of may cause the arthritis. But my opinion is not as important as the fact that it has worked — for generations.

I recommend the use of celery leaves (well washed) as well as the celery stalk, because the leaves are high in sodium. The stalk is high in potassium. The two together yield a sodium and potassium content five times greater than the calcium content.

The combination of organic sodium and potassium can react as a dissolver of those inorganic calcium deposits present in the body of a person suffering with arthritis.

Another benefit is the chlorine content which helps eliminate the waste material from the body.

Combining equal parts of carrot juice and celery juice gives almost a perfect mineral balance. If an arthritic takes this juice combination, it is frequently quite effective.

This preparation was used by two different men with quite advanced cases of arthritis. They both lived on farms in the same region of the country. Both experienced a decrease of approximately 50% of their pains within ten days to two weeks and also a greatly improved mobility of the shoulders and hip joints.

While millions continue to suffer from the crippling effects of arthritis, more and more of these sufferers are reversing the effects. These are the people who resist the use of powerful chemicals and instead combat the poisons that brought on the condition to begin with.

I know it's not popular to advise patients to give up something they like, but that is exactly what I am going to ask you to do if you have arthritis.

I am going to ask you to give up refined foods and go back to the natural foods you used to find in country kitchens. I am asking you that you give up sickly sweets, prepared mixes, and heat and eat types of pre-cooked foods.

If you continue to eat ice cream, refined white bread – enriched or not – cake, cookies, and candy, prepare to pay the price in arthritic suffering. It may be a bitter pill to swallow to give up these "treats" but *it is* the only "pill" there is to help alleviate arthritis.

Even the new cortisone drugs, the gold injections, the other new drugs that there never seem to be an end to, do not cure. All you are promised is the possibility of temporary relief. What you are threatened with, and not usually told about, are side effects that can be worse than the disease. Arthritis can cripple but it does not kill. But these chemical treatments can lead to fatal complications.

I admire the work of Dr. Giraud Campbell who is courageous

in his identifying the cause of arthritis in modern day diets and providing a regimen to reverse the effects — naturally.* He examines not only the intake problem, but also the problem of helping the body to get rid of these accumulated poisons via the skin, lungs, kidneys, and bowels, so as to restore normal functioning of joints. He must have had wise parents and grandparents.

I recommend you buy an electric juicer. Hand presses, though used successfully in the past, do not operate as efficiently. You will see your electric juicer pay for itself in the fewer fruits and vegetables you need to make the same volume of juice.

Vegetable juice is a concentrated remedy. My patients see quick benefits. You need mechanical help to juice a stalk of celery or a bunch of carrots. You help nature to help you.

Celery juice can be a blessing to arthritics. Combine celery juice with equal parts of carrot juice and arthritics can be twice blessed.

THE JUICE OF THIS COMMON VEGETABLE STRENGTHENS WEAK EYES

You do not usually consider poor eyesight as curable. Correctible with glasses, usually, but not curable.

Country people did not always have access to an oculist or optometrist. So they looked to nature. And nature made her cure so accessible even the blind could find it — carrots.

Carrot juice is an old-time remedy for faulty eyesight with a long standing reputation for measurable results.

A five ounce cup of carrot juice twice a day for two weeks brings definite improvement. Mr. L. was able to read lettering at fifteen feet that he could read only at ten feet before.

Frank E., complained of weak eyes. He complained that after reading the newspaper for five or ten minutes, his eyes felt tired. They burned and watered a lot. He recently had an eye examination and new eyeglasses were fitted. I found that he didn't care for and would not eat vitamin A type foods. He said he did like raw carrots but could not chew them properly on account of his dentures. So I suggested he drink six ounces of raw carrot juice with each meal. After only ten days of this therapy, Mr. E. re-

---

**The Doctor's Proven New Home Cure for Arthritis,* Parker Publishing Co., West Nyack, N.Y.: 1973.

turned to my office with a sparkle in his eyes and his complaints eliminated. He claimed he even had better distance vision while driving his car.

In my opinion carrot juice works because of its special vitamin A ingredient called carotene. This vitamin A is much more easily utilized by the body than the usual vitamin A concentrates that you get in vitamin A tablets.

Another reason that makes this vitamin A more compatible than a concentrate is that it is combined with vitamins B, C, and G and surrounded by a wealth of substances like potassium, sodium, calcium, phosphorous, chlorin, sulphur, magnesium, silicon, iron, and iodine.

Most of us have heard that carrots help you to see in the dark. This is true, but this is only part of the story. Carrots are helpful to your eyes day and night.

WRONG FOODS CAN MAKE YOU ILL, RIGHT FOODS CAN MAKE YOU WELL

Mom would never let me eat pickles and drink milk at the same meal. Nor would her Mom.

There are right combinations of foods and wrong ones. I have told you a few of my success stories. Here is one with a sad ending.

Mr. H., a former high school principal, was a patient of mine for several years. He came to me with the complaint of "heart trouble." Upon checking his blood pressure, I could find nothing drastically wrong. However, at certain times while listening to his heart it appeared to be laboring as if crowded by an excessive amount of gas.

I cautioned him repeatedly about his food mixtures, especially not to mix fruit with his principal meal of starches, which usually included potatoes, gravy, etc. He seemed to respond beautifully. Then I was shocked by a phone call one Monday morning from his wife. She told me that Mr. H. had passed away the night before. They had been to a church service on Sunday evening, and upon arriving home he had consumed a large dish of ice cream together with a large dish of fresh peaches. The cause of death was a coronary.

Improper mixtures of foods, of course, do not necessarily have such drastic results. The body has great natural wisdom and is able to come up with ingenious digestive answers to seemingly impossible problems that we give it. It is a chemical laboratory unequaled by anything that man has devised.

However, repeated disregard of compatible and incompatible food combinations can put a strain on the liver, pancreas, and other organs that supply enzymes and digestive juices.

A good food mixture is one that does not ferment during the time it is in the stomach. This fermentation is an important step in the manufacture of beer or whiskey. A cereal extract is combined with acids for a period of time to purposely cause fermentation.

Foods are either acid or alkaline. If acids are eaten with acids, the two form an acid mixture that requires certain digestive juices. This is easy for the stomach to produce. Digestion takes place.

When alkaline foods are eaten with alkaline foods, again digestion is an easy, natural process.

However, when an alkaline food is eaten together with an acid food, the two react together. The result is spoilage. The product of this reaction is an unnatural product which the stomach juices are not able to easily deal with. The result: indigestion, or gas, or lack of proper assimilation (absorption) of the original nutrients.

Common alkaline foods are sweets and starches.

Common acid foods are fruits.

High protein foods like meat, poultry, fish, and eggs, require a greater volume of digestive juices. They have an acid character. They should not be eaten with sweet desserts, but rather with fruits. Because they take longer to digest, observe this caution for at least four hours. This means that a between-meal snack after a meat or poultry meal should not be a sweet like cake or pie. Save that snack for after a meal that is lower in protein, if indeed you must indulge in a sweet like that at all.

Certain fruits do not mix well with certain vegetables, due largely to their acid or alkaline characteristics. Here are some common examples: Citrus fruit (orange, lemon, grapefruit) should not be eaten with watercress, cabbage, or turnip leaf; apricots not with green vegetables; prunes not with cabbage, onions, or watercress; carrots not with grapes; radishes and figs do not mix; nor do blackberries and beets.

Ebenezer who ran the country store never said a word to his customers about not eating the prunes he sold you after a dinner of corned beef and cabbage. He probably did not know. Most people in those days knew only about combinations they had trouble with or their neighbors or kin folk complained about.

So there was a lot of rumor and superstition about it, with many an argument cropping up over the cracker barrel.

We still have lots to learn today. People react in different ways to different foods. Gas for me, but maybe not for you. But if you go by the "acid and alkaline don't mix" rule, you are being good to your digestive system.

Use your own experience. If you don't feel your best an hour or two or three after a meal, remember the combinations and avoid them in the future.

Like pickles and milk.

WHAT WE ARE LEARNING FROM CHINA – SOURCE OF ANCIENT MEDICAL WISDOM

Recently, mainland China has opened for some travelers. American doctors were quick to take advantage of the opportunity, as China is recognized as one of the last original sources of natural healing methods.

Acupuncture is one example. Following the first visits in several decades, at which acupuncture methods were demonstrated in Chinese clinics, a rapid spread of acupuncture techniques took place in the United States.

This is a system of inserting needles into certain parts of the body to bring about certain results. Often the part of the body into which the needles are inserted bears no apparent relation to the symptom area. This is due to the network of nerve endings and meridian lines of energy that encompass the body and which Chinese doctors have grown to know intimately over the centuries.

Much of this work strikes a receptive note among chiropractors who find that pressures applied at certain points have beneficial effects seemingly unrelated to those points. More about this later. But it goes all the way back to Daniel David Palmer who in 1895, at the age of fifty, performed his first spinal adjustment on a man, Harvey Lillard, a completely deaf Negro who worked as a janitor in Davenport, Iowa.

When the treatment was over, Lillard reported he could hear. Following seven more daily treatments, Lillard's hearing returned to normal after seventeen years of deafness, and remained normal until his death years later.

D. D. Palmer was encouraged by this amazing case to develop his techniques and in the process founded chiropractic. Meanwhile medical men have laughed at Lillard's cure, saying there is no neural connection between the spine and the ears, and have given little respect to chiropractic founded as a result.

Today, the similar cures effected by acupuncture are tending to validate the Lillard story. It can no longer be swept under the rug by medical men. Thanks to the ancient art of acupuncture, the wisdom of those who have been here before us is more respected.

Foot reflex therapy is receiving a similar boost in respectability thanks to acupuncture. This is the foot pressure point therapy based on the supposition that nerve endings in the foot lead to all parts of the body. By pressing on special points in the sole or heel, you can stimulate a vital organ.

How can pressure on the ball of your foot help your stomach or your innards? We do not ask that question any more. We see a similar phenomenon in acupuncture, so we just remind ourselves we have lots to learn yet about the human nervous system and how it works.

AN UNUSUAL APPROACH TO CURING MALARIA

Recently I heard about an old Indian cure for malaria. It was purported to have been given to two young men about a quarter century ago by an old Indian woman who had a reputation for being a healer.

These two men were both suffering from malaria. She told them to sprinkle common table salt inside their shoes and to wear thin white socks. This they did. In one week's time their malaria symptoms disappeared and never returned.

Superstition? White magic? Placebo? Who cares, as long as it works. I have never tried it, only because malaria is not that common around here. But should I get such a patient, "Pass the salt."

If it works, there is a reason for it. Even if it is only the placebo effect, fine. This is the power of suggestion. You expect it will work because you are told it will, so the body obeys your mental instruction. Medical men often give sugar pill prescriptions, filled by the pharmacists with a straight face. You read the label, "Two every four hours". You take the pills. The symptoms disappear. Nothing wrong with that.

But I've got a sneaking suspicion that the salt cure has a different explanation. It may have something to do with those nerve endings in the foot. Or the salt may be absorbed by perspiring feet and get into the bloodstream. Maybe the malaria parasite cannot survive in a higher saline solution.

It goes back to why such old fashioned remedies as celery juice for arthritis work so well. There are other foods with high levels of these minerals. But these foods do not work as well as celery juice. What do you do, — skip the celery juice? Not if you've got the miseries. You take the remedy and ask questions later.

THE HEALING POWER OF GRANDMA'S FAVORITE TEA

"Hiram, have you noticed how good the cows look in the past couple of months — sleek, shiny coats?"

"Yep, Mathilda, and I know why. They've been grazing in that alfalfa patch."

Every time Hiram needed a tonic, Mathilda brewed some dried alfalfa leaves and made him drink a cup or two of the strong tea. It always helped him. Why not the cows?

In the 1956 issue of *The Herbalist Almanac*, published by The Indiana Botanic Gardens, alfalfa was given the following evaluation:

> After forty years of experience with thousands of botanicals from the world over, we believe no other single plant in the vast vegetable kingdom contains so many health giving properties as are contained in the alfalfa herb...The richest land-grown source of subnutritional trace minerals...more food minerals than any other land grown plant.

Are you listening, Mathilda and Hiram? You probably knew it all along.

Alfalfa looks something like clover. It is a legume and actually belongs to the bean family. Its secret may be that it sends its roots deep within the ground. Sometimes they descend as much as twenty feet. Here they find the precious minerals that other plants have already extracted from closer to surface soil. These minerals are stored in the alfalfa stems, leaves, and seeds, all of which then become valuable food.

One problem for humans is the taste — not exactly habit-forming. But alfalfa is now available in tablets. And, of course, the tea is around and when sipped piping hot is not at all bad.

The trace minerals found more in alfalfa than any other land plant are alkaline. Alfalfa is some ten times more alkaline than the average vegetable. This alkalinity helps to neutralize the acids of fatique and tension. Stiffness is alleviated. Kidney and bladder problems where acid is a factor are helped as is acid stomach.

Alfalfa is rich in pyridoxine, one of the B complex vitamins helpful to sore muscles and fatigue. Vitamin A is found in alfalfa in even greater concentrations than such prime sources as apricots or beef liver.

Thanks to another vitamin in this gold-mine of nutrients — vitamin E — alfalfa is helpful in adding strength to heart muscles.

I continue to hear reports of how alfalfa has been helpful for relieving arthritis, for lowering blood pressure, and for general body building where complaints do not necessarily point to a specific malfunction.

Surely alfalfa is one of nature's health remedies that deserves continuing use and appreciation.

NATURE'S CURES VS. CIVILIZATION'S RISKS

Nature seems to have supplied a natural remedy for whatever ails us. Yet millions continue to die of cancer. Is there a fruit, seed, leaf, bark, root, or vegetable waiting somewhere for us to discover, which can cure this disease?

Since it is pretty well agreed that cancer is a product of man-made civilization, perhaps that civilization will have to produce the cure.

A study by Dr. John Yiamouyiannis, Science Director for the National Health Federation, reveals that six cities with a population of over one million where the water supply is fluoridated have a cancer death rate some 24 percent higher than the national average.

Again, we have controversy over the benefits versus risks of this man-made change of nature.

Whenever I am asked to take sides in such a matter, you'll find me in nature's corner.

Dr. Theodor Reich of Switzerland, a leading specialist in medical statistics, has been quoted by the press as stating that people who live within one hundred yards of busy highways had a cancer death rate nine times greater than other people.

Little wonder we look skyward at the present fleets of jet planes and the possible advent of fleets of supersonic jets. Scientists warn that the exhaust from these supersonic planes can deplete the ozone covering in the stratosphere which protects us from harmful ultraviolet solar radiation. Are we inviting more skin cancer?

Yes, says Professor Harold Johnston of the University of Southern California who has been monitoring ozone depletion for the federal government. He estimates that five hundred supersonic jets, even with improved engines to reduce nitrous oxide emission, would produce 50,000 new skin cancer cases each year.

Recent studies throw some suspicion on the increased consumption of meat by modern man as a possible cause of cancer. Not only is there a correlation in the increase of cancer and of meat consumption over the past fifty years, but some findings also indicate a connection between the assimilation of animal protein and the formation of cancer cells.

"Mother Nature, what do we do now? Where is your remedy?"

"You created it, my boy; you remedy it."

Water is a good example. Up until about thirty years ago, city and country folk alike used natural soap made from vegetable oils and animal fats. Then chemical industry "blessed" us with something much less expensive and far more convenient — detergents.

Great. Mom was happy because the clothes looked cleaner. Dad was happy because the budget benefited. But something else began to happen.

Wells that produced pure water began to yield undrinkable detergent-filled water. Nature could purify water that contained natural soap, but not this chemical. Bacteria could change natural sewage into pure drinking water, but no bacteria were around that could work such magic with detergents. It was such a good chemical it would not degrade, or get reduced to simpler elements.

So in these areas where the water was being contaminated these detergents were outlawed. Also, man has now come up with new "bio-degradable" detergents.

He created it. He had to remedy it.

THE KEY TO REVERSING "INCURABLE" CONDITIONS

The old-time family doctor had one remedy that always worked. When he had no sure diagnosis or medicine to effect a cure, he'd say, "You need a change. Why not take a trip somewhere and get some rest away from everything for awhile."

The change seemed to always do the patient good. People came back revitalized, recharged, ready to go back swinging — and into the same trouble all over again.

Civilized life has created conditions that nature has no remedies for. So man must make changes in his civilized life if he wants relief from these conditions.

In December, 1966, the *Medical World News* reported the case of a 17-year-old boy admitted to John Hopkins hospital with hereditary nephritis. This is a kidney disease. Several years earlier his two brothers had been hospitalized for the same condition and both had died.

This time the doctors decided to put the boy on a special nutritive diet in addition to the usual monthly dialysis or blood filtering process. Within a short time he was out of bed and back home helping his father to harvest the tobacco crop.

It is ironic that this family was growing a crop, the mis-use of which is still killing thousands of people annually, while their children's kidneys were not able to handle the nutritionally depleted and chemically treated food they were feeding them.

However, the important point of this case is that a nutritional diet returned this kidney sufferer to a new level of health. Three other children in this family have now been put on this diet and are doing well.

Diet is usually the last thing that medical men resort to.

It should be, in my opinion, the first.

Perhaps it is not exactly accurate to call fresh produce, grown in rich soil naturally, nature's "cure." Prevention is a better word.

Malnutrition in the United States has been found to be more prevalent in middle and higher income than lower income families.

These are the people on the run, many of whom pamper themselves with rich foods. Rich foods eaten by rich people are not always rich in vitamins and minerals. The reverse is usually true. They are rich in sugar, starch, and fat.

A person can become overweight and still suffer from malnutrition. That is why so many dieters fail. They starve their body even more by cutting down on what few nutritional foods they may be eating.

A starved body is a vulnerable body.

Organic farmers have repeated the following demonstration a number of times: A patch of lettuce or other crop is planted in organically fertilized soil. The same type of planting is made nearby in a chemically fertilized soil. Not only is the growth faster and more abundant in the organic soil, but pests leave these plants alone while they attack in droves the weaker plants in the chemically fertilized soil.

Infection in human bodies gets a much more stubborn foothold where malnutrition exists. In 1965 The World Health Organization reported that when infection is coupled with malnutrition the results are far more dangerous.

The further we get away from nature's grandeur in our daily meals, the more vulnerable we become to functional disorders and disease.

THE SHOTGUN METHOD FOR COMBATTING INCURABLE DISEASES

There are many old-fashioned remedies that work on that principle. It is not so much that a special juice helps a special condition. It is more that you are giving your mineral and vitamin starved body a good dose of the nutritives it sorely needs.

The healing arts practitioner who favors natural healing methods may not know about the beneficial effects of celery juice for arthritis, but if he uses the shotgun approach, he can possibly be just as successful — the shotgun approach is, of course, blasting away with a high-powered nutritional program.

Nature is the source of this nutritional power.

Juicing fruits and vegetables concentrates this power even further.

Fruit juice and vegetable juice, freshly extracted, are loaded with nutrients that build the body's natural defenses.

So here are the rules to follow when you are faced with so-called inevitable conditions:

1. Cease intake of all civilized foods. This includes prepared foods, canned foods, and any foods with colorants, preservatives or other chemical additives.
2. Pause, to give your system a rest, before beginning your shotgun approach.
3. Use this day or so to rest and insulate yourself from mental problems, tension, or other worries.
4. Encourage better elimination with an enema.
5. Begin the shotgun nutritional diet, plenty of fruit juice and vegetable juice, raw vegetables, raw fruits, and only highest nutritional meats, like liver and other organ meats.
6. Maintain until symptoms are relieved. Add other foods, but avoid empty calories. This is nature's old-fashioned way of helping you to help yourself.

4

FOODS THAT INJECT VITALITY INTO YOUR VITAL ORGANS

If you were to go on a sightseeing tour of your body's internal systems, you would be attracted by several parts that occupy significant internal space: the heart, liver, kidneys, pancreas, and other vital organs, as they are called. If your sightseeing guide were to describe the services that these organs perform for you, you might stand a moment in a reverent respect before them and perhaps tip your hat as you left.

However, in real life, we observe anything but respect for these important organs. We don't eat natural foods right from the farms and orchards like folks did in the old days.

Instead, we eat foods that clog our "pipes" and put an extra load on our heart. We stuff ourselves with sweets and starches that make the liver and pancreas work overtime, and we consume chemicals and poisons in our food that never make it through our kidneys.

In this chapter I share with you the benefits of ancestral wisdom — ways to inject new vitality into lagging organs.

WHAT TO DO WHEN THE LIVER SLOWS DOWN

Mr. R. at 36 years of age should have been in the prime of life. But instead he was weak, run-down, logy, and looked 20 years older.

He did most of his work sitting behind a desk, yet, he said, he seemed to have not enough energy even for this. I weighed him in at 25 pounds overweight. He admitted he was a bread and potato man. This translates to starch and starch.

Upon examination I found a considerable amount of tenderness over the liver. I did not have to for a moment wonder why.

I put him on a special meat and grape juice diet, and asked him to come back in two weeks.

There were seven pounds less of him when he returned, pounds he could well do without. He said he felt more energetic and "full of life." I put him on the table. There was no longer any tenderness over the liver.

Let me tell why this diet is a boon to the liver. For a starch to be broken down and assimilated, a considerable amount of digestive juices are required, many of them supplied by the liver. A bread and potato person keeps the liver working overtime. Animal protein does not tax the liver for its digestion. In fact the acid in grape juice makes the meat easier to digest. Furthermore, the grape sugar, or grape starch, is in a form that requires much less work by the liver.

"But meat is so expensive," one woman complained when I advised this diet for her.

"More expensive than doctor bills?" I asked. No comment.

Another young, single woman flared up at the idea that she should take the time to cook a steak or roast or chicken just for herself. She prepared a quickie sandwich. I put her on the scale and pointed to the reading: "At 160 pounds and rising, how much time do you think you're going to be around doing things your way?" Again, no comment.

Sometimes you have to shock people into caring for themselves.

A word of warning: some people cannot go on this diet safely. They are diabetics. You may be diabetic without knowing it. So check with your doctor before beginning the meat and grape juice diet.

Now let me tell you the best animal protein and the best grape juices to use on this diet.

Poultry is animal protein, so is fish. There is less fat in most fish than you find in poultry. The skin of the poultry and the dark meat contain the concentration of fat. So if you stick to white meat and remove the skin, you are doing fine. Some poultry is just plain too fatty, like goose. Duck would have to be well-cooked, perhaps even over-cooked according to most tastes, in order to merit a place on this diet.

Put the same measuring stick on the meats you select and how you prepare them. Choose lean meats. Chopped beef is now offered by most supermarkets in various grades of fat content. You may pay a bit more, but it costs you less in the long run.

Veal is usually low in fat. But you have to be careful with lamb. Pork is just too fatty to deserve a place in this diet. Those breakfast meats, luncheon meats, and other types of sausages, franks, and spiced or smoked meats are to be avoided. Stick to the natural.

The best way to eat meat is raw, but few of us can enjoy it that way. Steak tartar (raw chopped steak) is served in some restaurants. Our forebears ate meat raw.

Priority methods to cook:

Bake or Broil
Stew or Broil
Fry

Frying keeps fat in and this type of direct contact with extremely high heats makes the meat less digestible. Grandma fried much less than we do today. She knew better. More time, but less heartburn. Today the deep fry is the mainstay of short order cooks, at the expense of our viscera.

If you have acute problems because of your liver, I would make the meat and grape juice diet your exclusive daily bill of fare — that's right — three times a day.

If you just want to be kind to your liver, have an occasional meat and grape juice meal. And, of course, there are all gradations in between the 3-meal-a-day diet, and the occasional animal protein and grape juice meal, depending on your liver's needs.

About the type of grape juice.

WHAT BACCHUS DID NOT KNOW ABOUT GRAPES

Grapes seem to have a significance for man.

Grapes appear throughout the Bible, and grapes and the juice of grapes, fermented or not, are used in many symbolic religious services throughout the world.

Whatever its esoteric values, the juice of grapes contains some very profound nutritional values. It is a source of:

Vitamin A	Calcium
Vitamin B1	Phosphorus
Vitamin B6	Iron
Vitamin B12	Copper
Vitamin C	Potassium
	Niacin

These are not only valuable nutrients for the body, but they occur in grapes in an easily assimilated form.

Of the many varieties of grapes available, I prefer the Concord grape which is the best known American grape and has been for over one hundred years. Our grandparents knew the Concord grape well, and used it as a remedy in many ways, even as a cold pack.

You will recognize the Concord grape by its deep purple color, as compared to the red grape or white grape. I don't know if the deeper color is connected with its more concentrated nutrients per fluid ounce than its less blueblood brothers.

There are about 120 calories to a six fluid ounce portion of Concord grape juice. About 95% of these calories are carbohydrate calories, but in a highly usable form, natural dextrose and levulos, giving the liver almost a free ride. The balance of Concord grape juice is mostly protein with a trace of fat.

If you grow grapes and have other red or white varieties, grape juice made of these grapes is fine. Use it. However, I do not consider the red or white grape juice you buy in the store as pure as the Concord grape juice, due to the additives that are usually required in order to retain color and flavor.

Bacchus looked at the grape as a doorway to revelry. Our grandparents looked at the grape as a body builder.

They used grapes to build up weak blood, otherwise known as anemia.

They used grapes to combat liver disorders, jaundice, and as a stimulant to bile secretion.

They used grapes as a mild laxative, as a dispeller of excessive mucus, as a nerve tonic, and as a stimulant to blood circulation.

Grape juice is probably one of the oldest and most successful diet aids, helping to burn off stored fat while at the same time keeping the patient from feeling low in energy due to low blood sugar.

I was visiting friends out on a rather remote Kansas farm recently, when the conversation turned to the health problem of a mutual aquaintance, John B. I told them the turn-about that came when I put this man on the grape juice diet.

"Did you send John a bill for that advice, Doc? My grandmother's been telling me about that for fifty years."

You will be hearing more from me about the benefits of grape juice later.

Stay on the diet for several weeks until you feel a definite improvement in your energy level and total well-being. Return then, to your normal diet, but strike off all that starch from your future shopping lists. Don't risk striking out.

A POWERFUL REMEDY FOR A TROUBLESOME GALL BLADDER

The gall bladder is a companion of your liver, often in sickness as well as in health. It is a small pear-shaped sac located under one of the lobes of the liver. It stores up bile which the liver produces, bile being a digestive juice that helps largely in the conversion of fats.

The gall bladder can become irritated or inflamed. It can also become clogged with stale bile and other pollutants. The usual symptoms are a tired feeling in the morning together with a feeling of nausea.

In the old days they put lemon juice in a bottle with a few other ingredients and called it a patent medicine. It was said to be good for summer complaint, colic, "green sickness," and wind in the stomach.

Of course the more thrifty among our forefathers saw through the label and squeezed their own lemons. The fact is, lemon juice does indeed stimulate, purge, and empty the gall bladder.

Take three tablespoons of undiluted, unsweetened lemon juice a quarter to a half hour before breakfast daily for one week, and notice the difference.

Cy J. was only 47 when he came to my office complaining of being "too tired and sick" to get up in the morning. It had been months since he could remember feeling the way he should. "I guess it's old age," he allowed.

"Nonsense," I replied, as I wrote out his lemon juice instructions. He called me the fourth morning at 7 A.M., sounding real chipper.

"I just wanted you to know how well I feel this early in the morning. That lemon juice works!"

I saw him again on the street, about six months later. He gave me a big smile and said that his early morning problems had never returned.

Lemon juice before breakfast is a powerful purge. You need to use it for only three or four days, but it may be used for a week or longer, if desired.

HOW TO WAKE UP IN THE MORNING FEELING YOUNGER

Many people wake up in the morning, get out of bed, and go about their business wondering why they feel so sluggish. One reason: their liver may still be asleep.

That tired, worn-out feeling is usually experienced by people in their forties and older, but I've seen many people in their twenties with "tired" livers.

Here is an easy way to massage your liver and wake it up. A naturally stimulated liver functions more efficiently. Everything feels easier for you. Instead of sinking into the deep mire of the "misery," you feel like you are floating through the day, and all's right with the world.

It is easy and brings such welcome benefits *(figure 4-1)*:

1. Place your hands on your lower ribs with your fingers spread forward.
2. Press the right hand in and then relax it.
3. Press the left hand in and then relax it.
4. Continue these alternate right hand, left hand pushes for 24 times.

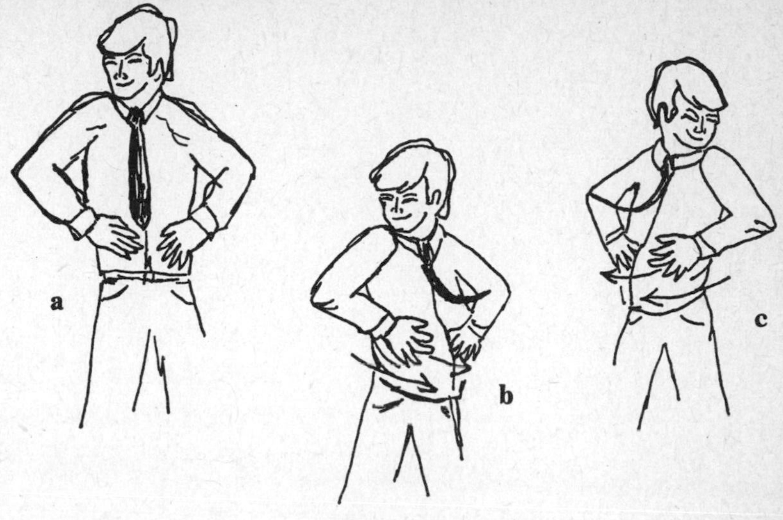

Figure 4-1

Liver Massage

The best position is standing. The best time is in the morning on arising. But, assuming your hands are free, you can give yourself this beneficial liver massage riding on the bus, walking to the store, or anywhere and anytime you think of it.

Henry J., 45 years of age, came to my office with a jaundiced complexion. It had progressed to the point where the whites of his eyes were a dismal yellowish-brown. He complained of having a heavy, tired, rundown feeling most of the time. It was quite obvious by his complexion that there was an over-taxation of his liver.

I checked with him regarding his diet. It consisted of too much of the wrong kinds of food, such as heavy starches and too many sweets, with no green vegetables.

Upon examining him I found a noticeable amount of enlargement of the liver with more firmness on the right side below the rib cage.

I demonstrated this exercise and asked him to try to do it at least once a day, preferably in the mornings upon arising. I also advised Henry to eat mostly green vegetables, eliminating the heavy starches and sweets.

Henry came to my office for about three weeks to be treated, during which time he also was doing the recommended exercise. It was gratifying to see how his complexion changed to a normal healthy color. The whites of his eyes cleared from their yellowish-brown to a normal white. His tiredness and sluggishness disappeared. The extra firmness below the rib cage on the right side seemed to disappear. Henry told me that this exercise was the best medicine he had ever used.

HOW YOU CAN HELP YOUR PURIFYING ORGANS TO CLEANSE YOUR BLOOD

On either side of your lower spine sit your kidneys, just at the rear of the abdominal cavity and slightly below the ribs. The kidney's main function is to collect the waste products of cell growth and cell replacement which collect in the blood and filter these out of the body in urine via the bladder.

Kidneys are subject to stones, tumors, inflammations, and other acute conditions. But more often they do not do the job efficiently because there is just too big a job to do. We load the body with foreign materials that have no place in our body and must be eliminated. The kidneys become sluggish under the heavy load, pretty much like your clothes washer would.

I have seen cases where medicines prescribed to assist the kidneys in throwing off an inflammation or to stimulate the kidneys into working harder only compounded the problem. They added one more poison to the backlog of poison needing to be eliminated in the urine.

Gerald K. came to see me with a kidney infection. He had been put on antibiotics. But they did not help. Usually when something does not work you try something else, but this man had been kept on the powerful antibiotics for two months.

I decided to turn the job over to nature and put him on a fruit and fruit juice diet which I'll describe to you in a moment.

Within a week Gerald showed a profound improvement. Within three weeks all evidence of edema, or swelling of the body with backed up poisons, was gone. He felt great.

Before you go on this fruit and fruit juice diet make up your mind, here and now, to eliminate further input of the poisons that are enemies of your body and especially of your kidneys. You know about them. But you partake of them anyway, figuring a little poison won't kill anybody. Don't be too sure.

A little poison can go a long way, if it becomes a way of life. Alcohol, coffee, tea and salt as a way of life can instead be a way of you-know-what. Let's talk about the poisons that confront us today, many of which our old folks never had to contend with.

MODERN DAY PROBLEM FOODS TO AVOID

Artificially colored, prepared, and preserved foods should be considered "a little poison." Did you ever read the labels on these foods? Some have as many as six or seven chemicals in them. None can be proved to be killers in the amounts used, but they all add up to health problems for those whose tolerance for these additives is low. And a common health problem they induce is kidney trouble.

Watch out for foods with the following chemicals in them. You won't suffer from eating them occasionally, but will probably have to pay in some way for making them a way of life:

Sodium nitrate
Sodium nitrite
Monosodium glutamate
Benzoate of soda
BHA
BHT
Sulphur dioxide

There are others. Read the labels. Our grandparents did not have to. They ate natural foods. If they had to preserve they stored in an out-cellar, a cool dry place they built for that purpose. Or they dried food in the sun. If they canned, they did not use preservatives except occasionally salt or sugar.

STARCH = FAT = A LOAD ON VITAL ORGANS

In a recent report to the American Society of Bariatric Physicians based on the study of 1200 adults selected at random, some 75 percent were found to be overweight or hypertensive (high blood pressure) or both.

Excess body fat comes from eating excess starch.

Starch, otherwise known as carbohydrates, is everywhere we

look. Sugar and sweets are carbohydrates, too. Heavy starch diets slowly rob us of our good health in at least three ways:

1. Starch causes fat to accumulate on the body, which becomes a strain on the heart, and on the other vital organs.
2. The digestion of starch taxes the liver. Eventually this organ rebels, the body becomes sluggish.
3. When excessive sweets are ingested, the pancreas is called upon to deliver insulin to the bloodstream in order to maintain a constant blood sugar level. An overworked pancreas can mean diabetes.

I wish it were only these three ways that heavy starch diets could affect us. You hear about these three ways most frequently because they are so defined and so cause-effect oriented.

Often the excessive starch causes more subtle imbalance in the system. When you get right down to it, there are few diseases or body malfunctions that a health specialist could unequivocably state could not have possibly resulted from heavy starch diets.

What foods are starch?

Cereals are starch. Like wheat flakes, corn flakes, rice flakes — all cold and hot cereals. This cake mix and that pancake mix, — all starch. So are cookies, crackers, candy muffins, marshmallows, pastries, pies, and pastas. Sweets like ice cream turns to starch. So do sodas and syrups.

Sound familiar? Were some people I know to eliminate these items from their daily menus, there would be little left.

Even fruits and vegetables are heavy carbohydrates. But these are nature-made, not man-made carbohydrates. With each fruit and vegetable carbohydrate molecule comes body nourishing minerals and vitamins. Depleted, denatured white rice, white sugar, white bread, tax the body, while raw fruits and vegetables build the body. Do you know someone born before 1900? Ask him.

OLD STANDBY FOODS THAT HELP YOUR KIDNEYS AND BUILD YOUR BODY

All fruits and melons were used as health builders by our forefathers, except highly acid fruits. Examples of excellent fruits are bananas, pears, apples, grapes, plums, avocados, prunes, apricots, cherries, and figs. Avoid the fruits that have considerable acidity. These include oranges, grapefruit, and indeed the whole family of citrus fruits. Peaches, persimmons, quinces are others.

Stew or cook other ways, if you wish, but never add any sugar or cornstarch when you do. Raw is still the best.

Melons are fine. Cantaloupe, watermelon, honeydew, cranshaw. Berries, too, with the exception of strawberries which are rather acid. Tomatoes are a fruit, but also too acid to have a place in this diet.

This exclusively fruit and fruit juice diet should clean out the kidneys in a few days even when the problem has been serious and of relative long standing. When you feel well enough to return to other foods, do so gradually, adding a few foods at a time, and watching the results.

If you are prone to kidney problems, take my advice, stay off those slow poisons I already mentioned and also avoid bread, rolls, pastry, crackers, muffins, cookies, pie, cakes, and other flour products.

Dairy products are different for some people's kidneys, and I often take my patients off milk, eggs, cheese, and butter.

Bill C. was a cheese hound. He also used globs of butter. Of course, both went on slice after slice of bread, toast, English muffins, and crackers. Bill suffered from aches and pains for so long he felt they were part of life. No more. I took him off these breadstuffs and spreads. He's now an apple hound and a healthy, pain-free man.

Vegetables are a good transition food once you return from the fruit diet to a more normal regime. One vegetable that is especially good for kidneys is asparagus. If you have ever urinated shortly after eating asparagus you know that even within an hour the rank odor signals the elimination of a large amount of body toxins.

Minimize the animal proteins at first. You will probably find that your body's tolerance for meat, fish, and poultry will be in direct proportion to the amount of physical activity your normal day includes.

A sedentary indoor life permits less protein than the active outdoor life. And be especially sure to avoid those proteins that are preserved — those cold cuts with the chemicals, chemicals that prolong the shelf life of the meat at the expense of yours.

The old-timers still stick by apple cider vinegar as a kidney remedy. I use it frequently for patients with sluggish kidneys and it is quite effective. I believe it is effective because of the potassium it supplies to the system. Potassium is often lacking to such a degree in our regular diet that kidneys cannot be adequately flushed. Also, vinegar supplies a natural acid that is helpful to the kidneys *Figure 4-2).*

Merely mix vinegar in six ounces of water. Use one teaspoon of apple cider for each fifty pounds of body weight. Drink three times a day, before each meal. Do this for two days, then skip four days before beginning again. These two days on, four days off cycles can be continued for as long as you feel it is doing you good.

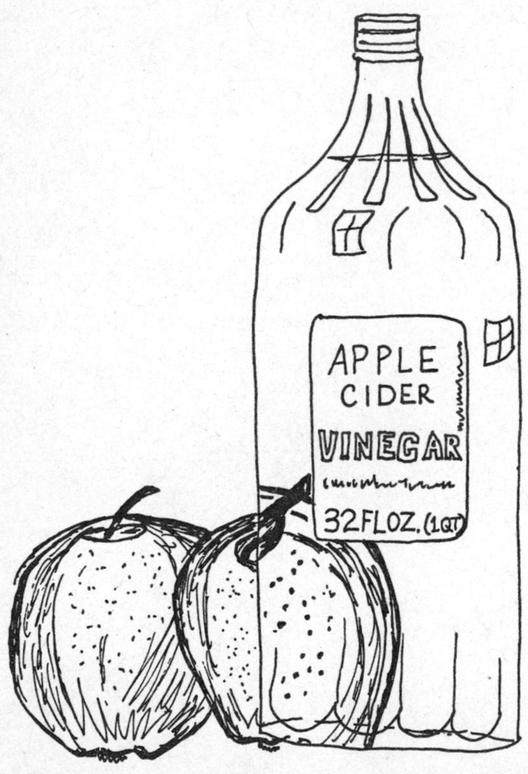

Figure 4-2

Let me put in a final plug for grape juice. Again, this great juice, especially of the purple Concord grape, leads the pack in therapeutic value to the kidneys. Its high iron content is a blood builder and the blood carries it to the kidneys where it promotes rapid healing of those irritated kidney tissues.

Irritate them no more. Be kind to your kidneys. You cannot afford not to.

THE BALMS YOUR HEART LOVES

Your heart loves everything your liver and kidneys love because when you help these organs to do their job, you help your heart, too.

To oversimplify, the blood pressure is one measure of the heart's proper functioning. High blood pressure usually indicates an extra load placed on the heart by blood vessel constrictions caused by tension or by blood vessel hardening or deposits as by cholesterol.

We know more about fat today than they did in the old days and know it can affect the heart, but they still had an intuitive reaction to it. People in Northern states tended to eat more fat, Southern, less. Eskimos can live almost entirely on fat, a diet which would soon clog our blood vessels with cholesterol. Clogged blood vessels put an extra load on the heart.

If you want to be kind to your heart, avoid animal fat, or limit it. Animal fat is our main source of the kind of fat that tends to form cholesterol. It is called saturated fat.

The fatty meats are beef, lamb and pork. Trim fat off before cooking. Trim each forkful before eating. When roasting or broiling, use a rack to allow fat to drain away. Spoon off fat from stews, gravies, soups, etc. by permitting them to chill first.

Butter is animal fat. Margarine is vegetable. Most vegetable oils are either polyunsaturated, meaning they tend to reduce cholesterol, or neutral, meaning they do not affect body cholesterol one way or the other. Corn, soya and safflower oils are polyunsaturated. Peanut and olive oils are neutral.

High quality protein foods that you should favor, if you want to favor your heart, are fish and poultry, both low in the kind of fat you don't want — saturated fat. Of course, avoid frying fish or chicken. Broil, bake, steam, or roast. Then when you take a forkful of poultry, remove the skin or fat globules.

Low blood pressure usually indicates a lack of heart vitality or low general body metabolism or rate of activity. It is this latter situation which we will consider now as it is more likely to be a circulatory system problem.

However, old fashioned remedies are not as specialized as modern medicines. Nature has a way of widening its areas of benefits.

For instance, whenever you see beets in your grocer's vegetable bins or at farms or in supermarkets, you see a heart balm *(Figure 4-3)*.

Our forefathers swore by beets and beet juice. Was this because it is red and blood is red? Or did they have more to go by?

Soloho is a Hopi Indian medicine man. As I write this, he is 77 and still caring for Hopis, Navajos, Apaches, and Zunis on reservations in Arizona and New Mexico. When he has a case of arthritis, sterility, diabetes, or other ailment to treat, he may not know just what herb or plant to use, so he prays to his spiritual

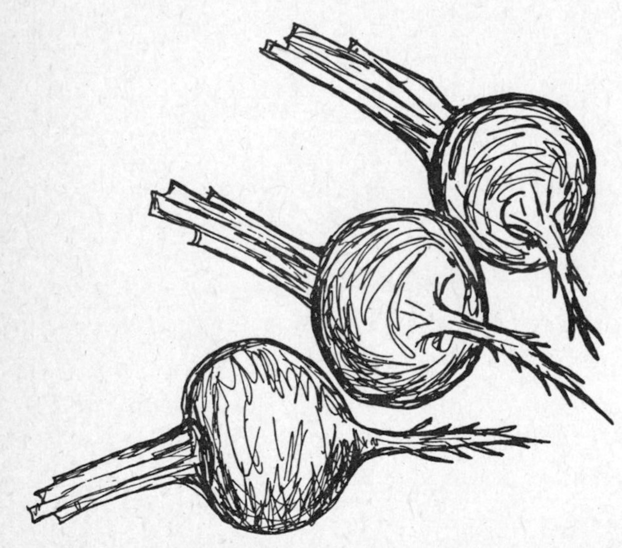

Figure 4-3

Red Beets – for heart balm

Father, goes out into the mountains, and then seems to know just what herb or plant is needed.

I am inclined to think that natural intuition, free of the influence of television commercials and newspaper ads, helped our forefathers to use certain foods for certain health problems and so to discover these natural remedies.

It so happens that modern analysis shows that beets have a high sodium and potassium content. They are thought to strengthen the fragile capillaries and thus restore weak heart valves and normalize varicose veins.

Other substances in red beets are silicon, chlorine, sulphur, magnesium, and iron. The list of vitamins they contain reads like the alphabet. Little wonder they also are recommended as a liver tonic, blood builder, and general tonic for the rundown body.

Diabetics should not use beets or beet juice before consulting their doctor.

Beets are very condensed nutrition. You do not go on a diet of beets, but merely add beets to your diet. One 6-ounce glass of beet juice plus one regular portion of beets a day should yield a noticeable improvement in lagging blood pressure.

Special advice to old people: if you feel cold in a room where younger people feel comfortable don't let them talk you into just putting a shawl or sweater on. Your body needs a higher temperature than theirs. Energy shortage be dammed — it's your life.

In the old days grandma pulled her rocking chair closer to the fire. Today grandma needs to turn up the thermostat. Doctors have found that even though an older person's hands may be warm or an oral thermometer shows normal readings, that person may be too cold to survive. The chest or abdomen area is the place to check. If the skin there does not feel warm, take immediate steps to warm the person. Old hearts need warm temperatures in which to function properly.

Finally we all need to remember that the heart is overloaded whenever we permit ourselves to tense up and react in fear or anxiety to life's problems and challenges. In later chapters, you will find many old-fashioned remedies that help to calm jittery nerves, get rid of the shakes, and restore peace of mind.

5

FOODS THAT PLACE YOUR BODY IN HEALTHFUL BALANCE AND MAKE YOU FEEL YOUNGER

Sometimes an old-fashioned health remedy does not work any more, like it used to. Take chicken livers. They were once looked up to as good tonic for the body because they were so rich in nature's vital foods. But today something new has been added to chicken livers that is not exactly good for you — arsenic.

Poultry farmers in the United States are feeding chickens arsenic compounds to help them grow faster. Maybe it works, but the livers of the chickens filter and collect this compound and so contain sizeable amounts.

Some ninety percent of all the chickens raised and about half of all the hogs are raised on these arsenic compounds. Result: Whereas the Federal Drug Administration allows .5 parts per million of arsenic in muscle meat and 1. part per million in edible by-products, pork livers on sale have been found to contain as much as seven parts per million of arsenic.

In the old days, you would not feed arsenic to chickens that you were going to be eating or selling to your neighbors. But nowadays, a few extra ounces on a chicken, no matter how attained, can add up to a lot of money when you produce tens of thousands of chickens a year.

Cross out chicken livers as a remedy, at least for now. But nature's resources are great, and she is still well ahead of man's interference.

NATURE'S REMEDY FOR AGING

Recently Dr. Linus Pauling, winner of the Nobel Prize in Chemistry in 1954 and the Nobel Peace Prize in 1962, reported to the International Academy of Preventive Medicine on his research to extend human life. He made five basic recommendations which, he said, would extend the period of productivity for the average person by as much as twenty years:

1. No smoking
2. Less sugar
3. Adequate intake of vitamins and minerals
4. Added daily supplements of vitamin C
5. Added daily supplements of vitamin E

Nobody can argue with the first three points Dr. Pauling makes, but the vitamin supplements have been controversial among medical men. So Dr. Pauling explained to the biochemists, physicians, and other professional people in his audience just why these vitamins work:

Free radicals in the tissues, he said, are the acknowledged cause of aging. These are incomplete molecular fragments produced in the process of oxidation, pretty much as a fireplace might yield a few bits of charred wood, incompletely burned. These radicals, he says, are troublemakers — like accidents looking around for a place to happen. Vitamin C and E, both antioxidents, help prevent their formation and, if formed, help to destroy them.

So vitamins C and E, supplied so richly by nature in certain foods, are like remedies for aging.

Perhaps if we led a more active life, we could eat enough of these vitamin C and E foods to delay old age. But our sedentary ways today make the vitamin supplements a more acceptable route to take.

I am not going to prescribe how many milligrams of vitamin C or E you should take. Nor will the minimum daily requirement spelled out by the authorities be of any help. You need minimum to survive, much more than minimum to thrive. And you may not receive any enlightenment from your doctor in this area where Dr. Pauling seems to be a lonely pioneer. Commonly, vitamin C tablets are in one and two hundred milligram sizes. Commonly, vitamin E tablets are in 100 international unit sizes. I'll say what the bottles say to you, "One tablet daily or as individually desired."

Try one tablet a day. Increase to two and see if it makes a difference in how more vital and energetic you feel.

Nature's sources of vitamin C are:

Green peppers	Citrus fruits	Strawberries
Cabbage	Rose hips	Brussels sprouts
Tomatoes	Broccoli	Mustard greens
Cauliflower	Melon	Dandelion greens

Nature's sources of vitamin E are:

Spinach	Meat
Turnip greens	Soybean oil
Eggs	Wheat germ oil
Seeds	Fish liver oils

Farmers have long known that animals with diet deficiencies lacked strength and energy. Their hair became dull and fell out Some had nerve debility and walked with aged gait. If this is so with animals, why not humans? And Dr. Pauling points the finger of suspicion to deficiency of two of Nature's life prolongers: vitamin C and vitamin E.

THIS FRUIT JUICE LAUNDERS YOUR BLOOD

In the last chapter I told you about grapes and the healing power they have for certain specific ailments. I discovered that the old folks were not being superstitious when they attributed a life-supporting faculty to grapes. I made this discovery the hard way:

I was hospitalized at the end of World War II with pleurisy and a collapsed right lung. Since that time I have had a lung tissue weakness, although I have regained the use of the lung. The grape juice diet is the means I have used to eliminate the mucus and phlegm which collects because of the lung's condition. I have remained on this diet for as long as seven weeks, feeling no ill effects and having more energy than I do normally.

I consider my own personal experiences with the grape juice diet little short of miraculous, as nothing else recommended to me had any such marked results.

There are many disorders that manifest in the form of excessive toxins of one sort or another. In my case, it was mucus and phlegm. In your case, it might be a loginess or aching muscles and joints or no energy.

Your blood may not be getting the cleaning it needs to get, which is the kidney's function. Too many impurities may be entering the bloodstream for a variety of reasons.

Whatever the reason, nature offers the beautiful grape to you. You do not have to squeeze the fruit, as the juice is readily available.

Here is how to proceed:

In severe cases, I recommend you consume nothing except undiluted, unsweetened grape juice, as much as you care to — for a period of three to four weeks. If desired, the grapes may be eaten in addition to drinking the grape juice.

In less severe conditions, I suggest the using of animal protein (meat) along with the grape juice. However, a diabetic should consult with his doctor before trying this diet.

The grape juice remedy seems to launder the blood. But it also seems to bring about other blood benefits.

Take the case of Mrs. G. I could see hers was an advanced case of emphysema. She was in her late sixties. I checked her breathing with a spirometer (instrument for recording exhalation). Five hundred cubic centimeters were the most that she could exhale. After being treated through chiropractic and placed on an exclusive grape juice diet, within one week she could exhale 2,000 cubic centimeters, a gain of 300 percent. Although this was not a complete recovery of her breathing, it was a remarkable improvement for so short a period.

Another case of advanced emphysema was that of a patient, a mine worker, 63, who had a distended abdomen because of "belly breathing." He faithfully followed the grape juice diet. He made rapid improvement in his exhaling, and showed a one-inch per day reduction of his abdominal measurements every day for a week.

THE ROLE OF THE LIVER IN YOUTH AND AGING

One of the functions of the liver is to manufacture and maintain the blood supply. This is a pretty important function and one which gives the liver a vital role to play in keeping us young.

In addition to this chief blood supply function, the liver has a few spare-time jobs like forming bile for use in digestion; preparing nutrients for absorption by the body; stimulating the elimination of waste, especially from the intestines.

It is also instrumental in the formation of urea, in the clotting balance of the blood, and in new cell formation.

Undoubtedly there are many other vitally necessary functions that we do not know about yet, but which together with the above add up to one very good reason why this fantastic organ is called the liver. It really "lives" us.

Take the matter of regulating the volume and quality of our blood. If this does not proceed as it is supposed to, you are a candidate for emphysema, edema, anemia, and many other degenerative conditions.

But there is one even more important reason to respect the liver: If it is not working properly, all the minerals, vitamins, and other nutrients you consume are not properly metabolized and instead of nutrients they become poisons in the body.

Without an adequately functioning liver, most of the old-fashioned health remedies — since they are based on the life energy in nutrients — are not able to work.

For that reason, I want to talk about ways to keep the liver happy. I want to do this before we leave the subject of food and get on other kinds of sly old secrets to better health that our grandfolks used.

The best way to avoid the miseries that a malfunctioning liver can bring down upon us is not to wait for signs of that malfunctioning and then try a remedy, but to treat your liver right starting today.

YOUR LIVER'S WORST ENEMY

Alcohol is one of the liver's worst enemies. Yet, it is often difficult to detect any problem until some ninety percent of the liver has been destroyed.

Alcohol destroys liver cells. The liver regenerates itself. In doing so, it produces connective tissue. This over-abundance of connective tissue ultimately results in the blockage of circulation through the liver and eventual liver failure.

Small amounts of alcohol are oxidized through perspiration, breath, and trips to the bathroom, but most of the task of burning off the alcohol falls upon the liver. Your liver is able to burn off between one half to three quarters of an ounce of 100 proof liquor an hour.

Suppose you have had five drinks in the course of an evening, — each drink being one and one half ounces of 90-proof whiskey or similar alcoholic beverage. It will take seven hours for the liver to return the alcohol-blood ratio to normal.

During this period the rest of your body is being affected by the alcohol. Like the toast goes: "Too much liquor ruins your liver, fuddles your brain, distorts your speech, cripples your coordination, and shortens your life span. So here's to masochism!"

The ingredient of liquor that does its dirty work is ethanol.

Ethanol is in many ways a drug. It affects the nervous system like an anesthetic, but not a very safe one. In large doses it is a killer. Used over an extended period of time it can damage the brain as well as the liver.

Forgetting the effects ethanol has on the higher brain centers that control judgment and just looking at the physical effects, ethanol dissolves the nerve cell fat, increases cell fluids, and temporarily inactivates the cells. The more you toss down, the more out of commission you go.

While at those non-physical levels, perception, reasoning, and intelligence go down the drain and we become at the mercy of instinct and emotion, ethanol has also anesthetized nerve reflex centers. At first, only muscle coordination is affected. But then comes loss of bladder and bowel control, loss of memory, and finally — loss of consciousness.

If enough liquor has been consumed, vital reflexes can also be affected — the muscles that control the lungs and the heart. Paralysis here can result in death.

HOW ALCOHOL AFFECTS INTERNAL ORGANS

There was always a bottle of whiskey around in the good old days. A swig right from the bottle gave grandpa a feeling of warming up.

Grandpa had a lot of good common sense, but here is one instance where he did not have a good hold on the old well handle.

Yes, small amounts of alcohol dilate the small blood vessels in the skin. This causes a feeling of warmth as a slight increase of surface blood flow results. But it is just a feeling.

In the rest of the cardiovascular system, there is a constriction of the vessels of the internal organs. This causes the internal body temperature to drop. Grandpa actually got colder, not warmer. His vital functions slowed down. His resistance lowered.

Now we know it is better to throw another log on the fire than to take a nip from the bottle. Liquor reduces body temperature and increases the loss of body heat through skin radiation.

Alcohol also causes nasal congestion and excessive use can cause lung congestion — another fallacy that the old folks had — hot toddies and brandy are good for colds. I was not around in those days, or if I was, I was too young to notice whether there was a devilish twinkle in Grandpa's eye. I just bet he knew better.

The reason frequent trips to the bathroom are needed by the drinker is due largely to the dehydrating effect of liquor on the body. All internal organs contribute to this outpouring through the kidneys. As resistance to disease goes down, metabolic imbalance goes up. A gradual diminishing of efficiency results. The heart does not exactly malfunction, but it does not function as well.

And as the heart goes, so goes the rest of the body.

HOW TO GET RID OF A HANGOVER

Jack B., in his fifties, had been my patient on and off for some ten years. Now he had come in without an appointment. I looked at him and could tell in a minute what his problem was.

"Jack, you are suffering from hypoglycemia, anorexia, acute gastritis, cellular dehydration, and anoxemia."

He gave me a murderous look.

"Wrong, Doc, all I need is something for a hangover."

Well, I could have offered him a Bloody Mary, or an Alka Seltzer, or onion soup followed by raw chopped steak. There are plenty of hangover cures around that don't work.

It is one of man's oldest afflictions. Pliny The Elder, a first century A. D. Roman, suggests in his 37-volume *Naturalis Historia* that the hangover be treated with "the eggs of an owlet... and the ashes of a swallow's beak, bruised with myrrh." Between orgies and such cures as these, I can understand the fall of the Roman empire.

Today, many cultures recommend "a hair of the hound that bit you." In Germany they stoutly maintain that there is nothing better in the morning than a cold bottle of double bock beer to put the world back into perspective. In Russia, it's a shot of vodka — neat.

In the United States, the old hangover favorites are Bloody Mary's and screwdrivers.

But there is another type of approach that you see in Europe and which some Europeans brought to our Midwest: salted cucumber juice in the Soviet Union, sauerkraut soup in Hungary — which evolved to sauerkraut juice or just plain sauerkraut here.

That's what I recommended for Jack. Sauerkraut juice mixed with tomato juice. I also rubbed his wrists and the back of his neck with ice cubes.

But I think what did the most for him was what I told him as he left.

"No charge."

Some years ago, I believe in 1966, an anti-hangover pill was introduced in Great Britain with some measure of success. It was called "Soba" and its active ingredients were largely B complex vitamins and a jolt of caffeine equal to two cups of strong coffee.

There is some validity to the use of these particular vitamins. Thiamine or B_1 supposedly aids carbohydrate metabolism and nerve function. Riboflavin or B_2 is helpful to the cellular oxidation process. And two other B-complex vitamins, nicotinamide (niacin) and pyridoxine in that British product aid in the dilation of blood vessels and in cellular functioning.

So when occasionally asked I say a good word for B-complex vitamins.

But still better words are "don't overindulge."

In summing up a "be kind to your liver" program, I endorse Dr. Pauling's five recommendations for longer life, and add one more to it — keep your intake of alcohol at a minimum.

THEY SAID "TEA IS GOOD MEDICINE" AND THEY ARE RIGHT

If you are not a drinker, you are said to be a tea-totaler. That has nothing to do with "tea" but I am going to connect the two.

A kettle of tea was always on the stove and while the men folk may have preferred that nip from the bottle, the woman folk had their tea.

And the women lived longer than the men.

I don't say the difference was necessarily the tea, but tea does make a difference.

We talked about herb teas a while back, but plain ordinary tea is also a long-time remedy that will continue to be around for a long time still.

The common variety of tea is made from the dried leaves of a shrub of eastern Asia called Thea Sinensis or Camellia Sinensis. Steeped in boiling water, the resulting beverage is getting new respect and recognition by researchers.

At a seminar sponsored by the New York Academy of Sciences, tea was cited as good for headaches that are due to hypertension. It was also described as soothing to the stomach.

Proponents of natural hygiene like Dr. Paul C. Bragg,* noted life extension specialist who is 94 years young and going strong, would argue with the health benefits of regular tea. It contains tannic acid used in making leather. No wonder it desensitizes the stomach, Paul Bragg might say.

University of London researchers have reported that tea reduces the build up of cholesterol in the blood vessels. Since this could add years to your life, this goes even further than the

*Robert B. Stone, *Paul Bragg: The Man Who May Live Forever,* (New York: Simon & Schuster, 1977).

kitchen stool experts would dare to go, and they have been proclaiming the remedial powers of tea ever since pre-Colonial days.

Russian doctors treat miners suffering from the intense heat of coal mines by having miners drink hot tea. In many countries tea leaves, moistened with warm water and placed in a gauze bandage, are used as a poultice to combat infections.

Were I to argue against tea as a remedy it would be like talking against motherhood. A cup of hot tea can be a good bracer. It has some beneficial minerals and, blessing of blessings, no calories. But...

You do not benefit by taking remedies as a way of life. Drinking tea and coffee indiscriminately can bring on a host of unwanted conditions that they themselves won't remedy; remedies for the effects of these stimulants may not be that easy to discover. So — moderation.

A POOR MAN'S GUIDE TO REMEDYING HEALTH PROBLEMS

A woman seeks medical help for a painful thyroid disorder. The first doctor listens to her symptoms and prescribes X medicine.

There is no improvement, so she goes to another doctor. He checks her, listens to her complaint, and based on the symptoms he considers indicative of the problem, he prescribes Y medicine.

After no improvement from this medicine either, the woman tries a third doctor who concentrates on different symptoms. The woman goes through the same disappointment with a third medicine, Z.

Then she hears about a doctor who practices a different kind of healing. He looks at the body as a work of nature, an organic unit with all aspects of itself interdependent. She decides to go to him.

He practically ignores the symptoms. Instead, he looks at the overall condition of the body. Is it toxic? Is the acid-alkaline level in balance? What about muscle tone, blood pressure, elimination?

This holistic view of the body from all angles is not likely to point to the need for any chemical. It is more likely to point to the need for a change of diet, massage, special movements, hot or cold applications, aids to better elimination, and other means for total body rehabilitation.

Folk medicine used this approach. It was highly successful. Of course, if adopted today, it would severely cut into the income of medical practitioners, so in a way I don't blame them for hitting out against vitamins and minerals and blasting old-fashioned remedies as superstition.

I am not saying that you should abandon standard medical care. What I am saying is that while you attend to symptom treatment, you should remember to give your whole body a chance to exercise its own recuperative powers.

This is the last chapter that I am going to devote entirely to foods as remedies. Foods are probably your best remedies, but not the only remedies that nature has offered us and which our forefathers had the wisdom to recognize.

In the chapters ahead I am going to reveal some old-fashioned remedies that have gotten lost in the attics and buried in the cellars of our grand-and-great-grandparents. They were shunted aside only because medical practice came along with some remarkable medicines and "miracle drugs."

But now people are having second thoughts. The hospitals are full. Medical expenses are taking a bigger and bigger slice of the family income. One illness is cured and another is incurred.

So they are dusting off some of these old remedies.

For me it is like an old family reunion, because I have always respected these natural means of treating the whole person and used many of these in my practice as well as in my own home.

Now I don't feel quite as alone as I used to feel.

Part of this new appreciation of natural remedies is evidenced in the home gardening trend. People are planting fruit trees and vegetables no matter how small their back yard. Even apartment dwellers are finding ways to grow chives, tomatoes, lettuce, parsley, and other vegetables in pots and flats.

People are sprouting mung beans, alfalfa, and soy beans in their kitchens and using these sprouts in their salads.

People are growing lemon trees in pots and harvesting beauty as well as nutrition.

People are growing angelica for rheumatism, mint for stomach problems, and aloe for burns — all on their porches, patios, decks, verandas, even window boxes.

Ten feet by ten feet can be a good size garden in which you can grow carrots, beets, cucumbers, and other remedies I have and will discuss in this book. It takes little time and hardly any expense.

Some municipalities are making park land available to taxpayers who wish to stake out gardens. There is even Federal funding for community action programs that include growing vegetables on available land.

This is great. I applaud it. And I don't just pay it lip service, I grow fresh vegetables at my place.

Old-fashioned ways are thrifty ways. Old-fashioned remedies make good common sense. Old-fashioned-health care used nature as doctor and nurse. How much more professional than nature can you get!

6

LITTLE THINGS THAT YOU CAN DO THAT PAY OFF IN HEALTH DIVIDENDS

Did you ever see Grandma do setting-up exercises?

Did you ever hear of Grandpa jogging at any time in his life?

Did you ever hear of any old folks from the days before so-called modern ways lift dumbbells or use exercise equipment?

No, you did not. Dumbbells are well named. In the old days, you would not dream of putting physical strains on your body by such strenuous activity.

Motions were gradual and productive. Grandma strolled. Grandpa rocked. It got her where she wanted to go. It gave him a feeling of motion through his body, too.

Motion is part of the old-fashioned way to physical fitness. Exercise came later. And sometimes when I look at some of the physical stresses and strains to which people subject themselves, I wonder if it should have come at all.

Again, let's take a look at nature. Old faithful. Do you see dogs doing calisthenics? Or cats? Oh, they get playful at times.

That's good. Gramps tickled the old lady sometimes and she threw a cushion occasionally at him.

But what you see animals do is stretch. And yawn.

HOW TO WAKE UP TO A BETTER DAY

Watch your cat next time it gets up from a snooze, or your dog.

First the front paws are stretched out, then the back. The whole torso is elongated. Then a yawn. And another stretch.

What is really happening?

Seldom does a person analyze what is really taking place through this stretching and yawning procedure.

The old folks got up early in the morning. Sometimes before dawn. Theirs was a long day, but that does not mean it was a hurried day or harried.

Today, the alarm rings. We pop up, dress, wash, gulp instant juice, instant cereal, and instant coffee and we're on our way.

Hey, come back. ("Who me?") Yes, you. You forgot to stretch and yawn.

That sounds silly. But it was not silly a hundred years ago. Turn back your alarm clock to five a.m. and your calendar to 1877.

Grandma is waking first. She's stretching her legs, now her arms. Now she's yawning. She sits up, puts her feet on the floor. Now she's surveying the situation. The old man's still asleep. She'll give him a few more minutes. Now she bends back with her hands on the back of her neck, arching her back. It feels so good, she's wiggling her toes. Here comes another yawn.

Now she's up and about.

A few minutes later when the old man arises, it sounds like out in the jungle. He roars, wheezes, coughs, blows his nose, and roars some more. Meanwhile, as he clears the respiratory system for action, he's also getting the blood moving in his arms and legs, first by stretching pretty much like Grandma did; but then he throws in a few slaps and stomps for good measure.

Both of these people were doing what comes naturally *(Figures 6-1, 2, 3)*.

But it does not come naturally any more. We have substituted for nature in so many ways, we have not noticed that a natural morning start has drifted away and we have put nothing in its place.

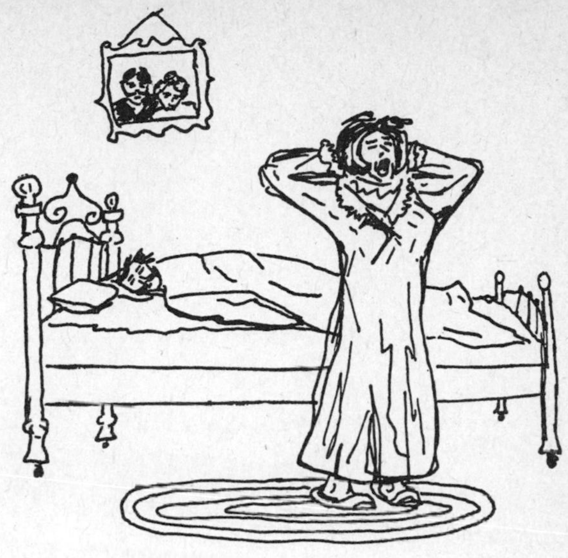

Figure 6-1

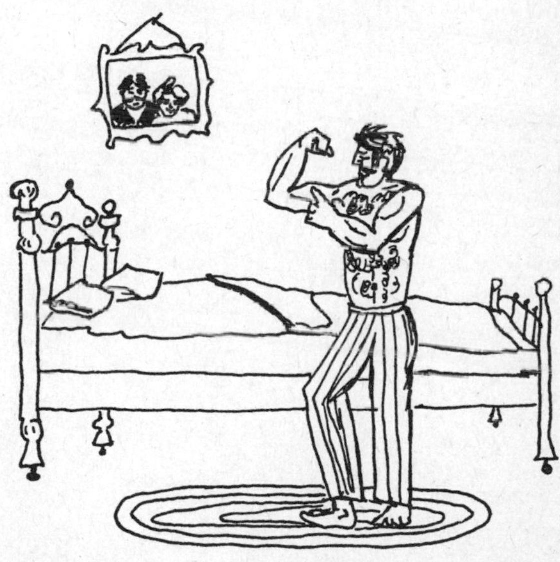

Figure 6-2

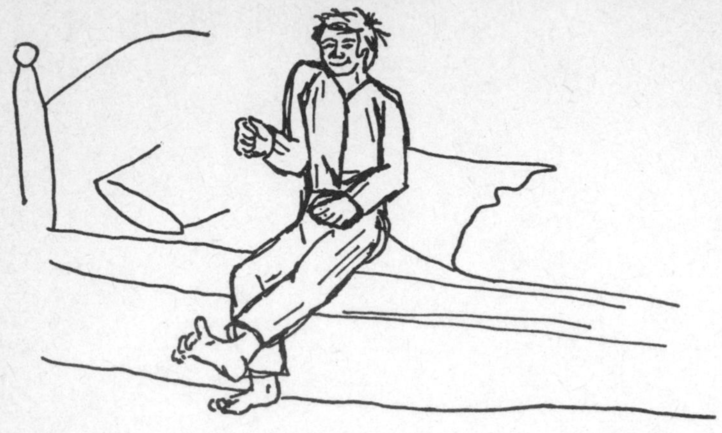

Figure 6-3

We treat our car better. We wait until the oil pressure gauge shows normal, and we idle the motor a few moments before stepping on the gas.

Paul G., 35, was beginning to wonder if old age was singling him out prematurely. He hated to get up, had no appetite for breakfast, dreaded walking into that office and having to function at his desk.

There was nothing organically wrong with Paul that I could see. I told him he had a sluggish system and that he had to spend a few minutes waking it up in the morning.

"What should I do?" he asked.

"Just stretch and yawn," I replied.

That's courageous for a doctor to tell a patient. No special exercises? No prescription? But Paul was a good sport and he gave it the old try.

Now it's a way of life for him. Stretching and yawning did so much to liven up his day that he has "adopted" it as his waking up routine. "Adopted" was his word. "Restored" is the one I prefer.

We need to restore nature's wake-up toning for our own body. In case you have forgotten how here is one way:

1. On awakening and prior to arising, force a yawn by

opening the mouth wide and pretending to yawn. The first try usually triggers a genuine one.

2. Now stretch the legs, actually making them longer.
3. Reach the arms upward toward the ceiling. Try to reach the ceiling.
4. Place your hands behind your head, fingers locked, and push your head backwards against your locked hands.
5. Return your arms to your sides and rock gently from side to side.
6. Place your feet on the floor and take a deep breath in the sitting position, exhaling slowly.
7. Move your shoulders around.
8. Wiggle your ankles and toes.
9. Stand up. Place your hands on your face, permitting the fingers to gently clean around the eye aperture.
10. Get going.

Yawning relaxes the muscles of the heart and accelerates the flow of oxygen from the lungs into the bloodstream and, of primary importance at this particular moment, into the brain. For some strange reason, yawning is an involuntary action that is very easily triggered. Watching someone else yawn can start a chain reaction in a room. As I suggested above, just by pretending to yawn, you can induce the real thing. Just by thinking about yawning you can feel a yawn coming on.

Go ahead. Yawn. I'll understand.

HOW THE WAY YOU STAND CAN MAKE OR BREAK YOUR DAY

In the old days men were men and Casper Milquetoasts wound up in the comic strips. One of the first things that struck the awakening man was his duty to be the strong, protective member of the family. So he reflected this self-image by standing tall.

Today men are usually the providers more than they are the protectors. They bear the load of financial responsibility. They remember this when they get out of bed and stand all stooped over with these burdens.

Women have succumbed less than men to this poor morning

posture, but they would do well to borrow a page from this chapter, too.

Take Morton H. He had chronic constipation and headaches. His middle-aged looks belied his youthful age of 34. He was married, two children. He ran a hardware store.

"How long have you been in business?" I asked him.

"Since my father died ten years ago. He built the business up. I've got all I can do to keep it going."

Morton looked like a candidate for future back trouble. He was stooped over from the burdens of the world. I asked him to stand erect.

He tilted his head up. He had forgotten how. I had to back him against a wall and show him how. "All parts of your back — hips to head — touching."

Somehow when a person stands up straight, his outlook changes. Morton seemed to feel this instantly.

Being weighed down by the world stoops a man. Then as the stooped posture becomes habitual, even good days disappear. Straighten up and optimism flows back in. It's like the tail wagging the dog.

Morton was smiling, something I did not normally connect with him. I just knew there could be a change. He called me a week later. Energy flowed through him. He felt more alive. His bowels were normal and the headaches were gone.

Have you looked at yourself in a full-length mirror lately? Take in your front, back, and side views. If your house has no combination of mirrors that permit this, drop in to your local clothing store and try on a new dress or sports jacket. But leave the store with a new, more erect posture:

- Neck vertical
- Shoulders flat
- Backbone straight

A stretching that is good for posture which you can add to your morning getting up fun is done lying on the floor face down. Reach your hands as far beyond the head as possible. Reach as far down with the toes as possible. Now arch the back.

Early in this century an Australian man named Matthias Alexander began teaching a method of re-educating the body to its natural stance and state. Today, The Alexander Technique is taught by hundreds of specially trained people in Europe and America.

The special command of these teachers is, "Let the neck be free to let the head go forward, to let the back lengthen and widen." Students of the method mentally repeat these words with the teacher as they stand, lie, sit, and move. The teacher does not treat and in fact hardly touches the student. But changes occur in the body through this learning process — not only changes in posture, but changes for the better in health.

Negative thoughts affect the body. Then the body tends to perpetuate the negative thoughts. You need help to break that kind of cycle — to help you out of the rut.

Chiropractic is giving that kind of help every day. Ours is a more physical approach, but we appreciate the mental factors, too.

You may want to seek professional help to "straighten" yourself out. Nine chances out of ten you can help yourself to make a great improvement in your posture by seeing the problem in a mirror and consciously making a change, little by little.

Be aware of how you are standing, sitting, and walking.

If your way is apart from nature's way, you know who moved.

A SPECIAL WAY TO "HANG TEN"

As a child I once saw an old man step on a chair, reach up and grab a rafter, kick away the chair, and just hang there by his hands. I remember I thought it looked like great fun. So when he dropped himself to the floor, he picked me up and let me do it. Of course, I looked down, panicked, and he had to lift me right down.

Later, studying chiropractic, I learned that what the old man had been doing was in the nature of a remedy. It was a way of stretching that we talked about earlier in this chapter.

Open rafters are no longer a part of modern home design. So when I decided I wanted such a place in my office I installed a pipe at the right height to make this hanging and stretching convenient not only to me but to my patients.

Occasionally, I would get questions about the purpose of the pipe. "I use it to hang myself," I would say jokingly and, if I was in the mood, I might demonstrate.

However, I started to get some strange looks. Patients would eye the pipe uncomfortably. When some stopped coming to me, I decided to remove the pipe. I installed it in my basement where I could still enjoy its benefits without alarming anyone.

A metal bar, which is firmly attached within a door casing or other sound structural members, is probably one of the most profitable investments you can have in your home. The benefits you can derive from this bar I believe are nothing short of miraculous. Through its proper use, the muscles can be extended in the arms, shoulders, back, and rib cage. Your body, as nature wants it to be, is restored.

I do not recommend that you chin yourself. Instead, grip the bar firmly with both hands, and allow yourself to hang freely from this bar, as long as you can hold your grip and still feel relaxed. Do this stretching twice a day, in the morning and in the evening.

This helps a number of complaints, as well as prevents them. Mr. R. complained of soreness throughout the middle and upper part of his back and shoulders, with numbness in his hands and arms. He did not rest well at night. These complaints made it difficult for him to do his work as a carpenter.

I instructed him to exercise at home by grasping his hands on an exposed overhead water pipe in his basement, then bending his knees, so his weight was carried by his hands and allowing his body to relax. After one minute of this stretching position, he was instructed to stand up on his feet and relax his grasp. After two weeks of this daily home therapy, his symptoms disappeared.

In surfing, there is an expression "hang ten." It means to stay upright on a board, riding a wave, for ten seconds.

I say "hang sixty." Sixty seconds a day of hanging can do wonders for your youth and vitality. Remember how Tarzan was pictured swinging on vines and from tree to tree? Well, I'm not going to get into that debate about man descending from the apes, but I'd be willing to wager nature once counted on our hanging to overcome the stresses of gravity. And maybe still does.

No wonder they built homes with open rafters in the old days.

HEALTHY TIPS IN YESTERDAY'S DAILY LIFE STYLE

My parents, and their parents before them, grew up in a home where walking five to ten miles a day was natural. In addition, children climbed trees, skated and sledded in the winter, helped with the farm work in the summer.

They went to bed early, and got up early. I used to hear "It's the sleep that you get before midnight that helps you the most." And wasn't it Ben Franklin who said, "Early to bed, early to rise, makes a man healthy, wealthy, and wise"?

I am more inclined to agree with Ben's homey health philosophy than Mark Twain's sarcasm: "The only way to keep your health is to eat what you don't want, drink what you don't like, and do what you'd rather not."

I don't believe in eating and drinking what you do not find to your taste. Everyone is different and nature gives us tastes to suit our special needs. I'm not talking about sweetness. Sugar clouds the issue. I'm talking about the taste difference between a steamed potato or steamed rice, between a can of salmon and a can of sardines, or between a raw apple and a raw pear.

Enjoy what you eat. Enjoy what you drink. Enjoy what you do.

Most people just do not enjoy doing calisthenics. I say don't do calisthenics. Instead, do whatever kinds of activity you enjoy.

There's a man and woman I used to see walk around their back yard a certain number of times every morning and evening. You could count on seeing them like clockwork — he striding in front, she following behind him. So mechanical. So synthetic.

It would be different if they held hands. Or if they stopped to yank out a weed or smell a flower.

Then there are the joggers. They run nowhere for running's sake. And the weight-lifters, pusher-uppers, and one-two-three'ers of all sorts.

Our heart, an incredible mechanism, pumps two thousand gallons of blood through our circulatory system a day, though it weighs less than a pound. When we exercise strenuously or put it under stress, our heart can pump ten times its normal volume. But nature has provided this factor of safety for use in emergency or survival situations.

Nature has a purpose in everything. Stretching feels good, yawning, too. Standing up straight makes you look good to the world and the world look good to you.

Walking is the best exercise there is. But walking for walking's sake is unnatural. Walk to get from here to there. Walk with a purpose. Walk instead of ride sometime, just to feel closer to the place you live or work. Walk briskly when circumstances call for briskness, not just for the sake of a fast tempo. Stroll when circumstances are right for strolling. It does not matter, just so long as you are flowing with nature, in consciousness as well as in body.

Do you feel energetic? Then let your arms swing and walk jauntily. Do you feel joyous? Then let your body express joy as you walk. Are you strictly business? Then walk in a businesslike way. Be as you walk.

When people become sedentary in their ways, a lot more likely today than a couple of generations ago, arteries become clogged from disuse. Postal workers who deliver mail have been found to have a lower incidence of heart attacks than those who work on the same mail inside post offices.

Moving around increases the need for blood in the voluntary muscle fibers and the network of capillaries that surround them. Movement also causes blood to be squeezed out of capillaries and into the veins, making room for fresh blood from the arteries.

A person who has moved around for a half hour has a lower blood pressure than when he started. That is because the blood has been forced into more capillaries, making more room for the blood supply.

When this blood is able to flow through capillaries that were previously clogged, the capillaries soften and become more efficient carriers of blood nourishment to the body cells they serve. Can't you just hear these cells rejoice?

We are geared to such an exhausting mental pace these days, we need to remind ourselves of some of the simple rules of healthful physical living that were part of our forbears' life style.

They ate well for both health and enjoyment.

They worked hard yet they relaxed, too.

They walked and they made every step count.

Most remembered the Greek philosophy of nothing in excess and they were moderate in the things they did.

It is questionable whether they remembered the Chinese philosophy of seeking advice to keep well instead of waiting for illness and then curing it. But then wasn't it somebody's grandmother who has been quoted all these years?

"An ounce of prevention is worth a pound of cure?"

OLD-FASHIONED MIND RELAXERS THAT STILL WORK TODAY

"Need rain."

"Yep."

That is an entire conversation between two farmers passing each other near the general store.

The crops are dry. Their very life depends on those crops getting rain. But no use talking about it or worrying about it.

Today we worry. We are the most prolific worriers in history. We have perfected worry and made it a science.

And it is a murderous science.

Worry is a killer. When life went at a slower pace there was less to worry about. Worry stood out more – like a sore thumb. If somebody started to worry about something, it would not take but a few seconds before they'd hear, "Worrin' ain't gonna do any good."

Today, if you don't worry you stand out in the crowd. The person who is calm and philosophical gets on other people's nerves.

But he lives longer.

Young pioneer couples watched the sunset together. Fifty years later they were still watching sunsets together. Were they really watching the sun go down? Yes, but behind that was a deeper purpose. It was symbolic of the end of a day of activity.

It was the time to relax.

We still have sunsets. But we no longer have the time to watch them. This, too, is symbolic. It reminds us that we no longer take the time to relax.

A farmer also sat down and looked over his crops. Was he thinking? Maybe? But I'll wager he was also not thinking. Just "settin'." Maybe he even had his eyes closed.

Remember how Grandma often dozed off while crocheting? Or Grandfather started snoring in front of the fireplace?

These were the rocking chair days when relaxing was the science, not worrying.

Take a few tips from these people:

- Think about good things that could happen. Do this especially whenever you find yourself worrying about bad things.
- Take one half minute occasionally during the day to close your eyes and forget the world, letting your mind go blank.
- Watch a sunset, a sunrise, a stream, a rain shower, interesting clouds, or other activity of nature at least once a day. Or, if you are not in a place where you can do this, close your eyes, take a deep breath, then picture such a scene of beauty and tranquility in your imagination.

Old-fashioned ways to relax are still effective today. In the days before contract bridge, people played checkers and dominos. Some played chess. I've seen people get up from a bridge game livid with rage at their partner — a bundle of nerves. I never saw a nervous game of checkers, and in chess you could fall asleep in between moves.

Tension is a killer. We need to take steps to remove tension from our daily life. We need to inject periods of letting go into our schedule.

Folks south of our border and in southern Europe still take a mid-day siesta. A nap is a perfect way to head off tension before it can get a hold on our ligaments, nerves, and vital tissues.

After tension has got hold of you, then it is practically impossible to reap the benefits of a snooze. However, if you know a couple of tricks you can come close and coming close to taking a nap can be a real boon to tense and frazzled nerves.

- Take a few deep breaths. Slowly.
- Yawning helps. Induce yawns.
- Start at one hundred and count backward slowly.

Even if you do not fall asleep after taking these three steps, you have helped yourself to a healthy portion of relaxation.

MASSAGE AS RELIEF FOR BODY INFIRMITIES

The body rub is one of the oldest of health treatments. It feels good, because it is good.

Most people today relegate massage to the massage parlors, Turkish baths, and spas. But you can give each other a healthful massage at home. You can even give yourself a massage, though less complete.

The professional masseur or masseuse, the chiropractor, the physiotherapist of any discipline needs to have thorough knowledge of anatomy. There are schools of massage in Europe where the courses of study include physiology, bacteriology, histology, diagnosis, and hygiene.

Although massage probably goes back to the beginning of the human race, it is first mentioned in Chinese literature some 3,000 years B.C. Then, Hippocrates, the early Greek physician, used massage with good results.

The Samoan slap dance is said to have originated as a self-massage. Today, we recognize massage:

- Increases blood supply to the cells
- Improves digestion
- Develops muscles
- Stimulates elimination
- Actuates vital organs

There is hardly an area of the body that is not benefited by massage. It is hard to understand why people are forgetting about massage, especially the home grown variety.

The professional knows just how and where to rub, squeeze, knead, knuckle, vibrate, and slap. You do not have to know these techniques to provide a beneficial massage at home to parent, mate, child, or self.

Let's start with a few sinple self-applied hand movements that make your cells feel better *(Figure 6-4, 5, 6).*

1. *Face massage.* Take both hands and palm your cheeks and eyes. Now gently move hands backward towards ears. Repeat a few times, applying pressure only to the degree that it feels good. Special dividend: Good for removing wrinkles.
2. *Hand massage.* Crack the knuckles of each finger by gently pulling. Wring your hands. Feel them tingle with increased circulation?

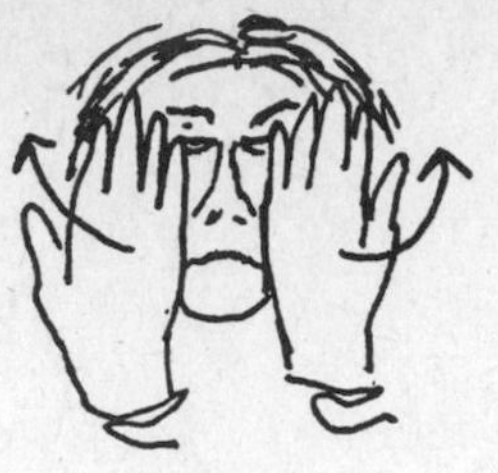

Figure 6-4

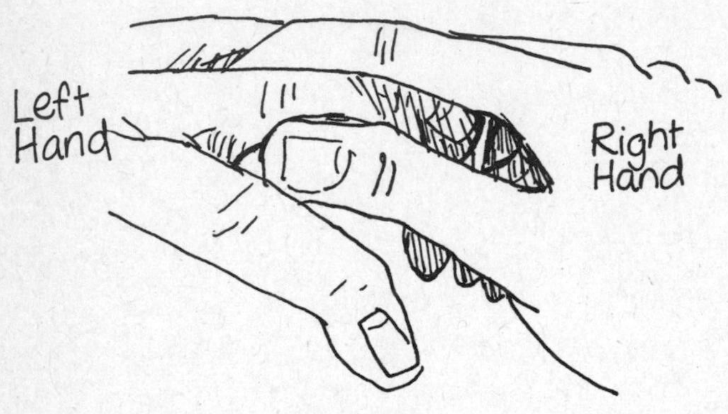

Figure 6-5

3. *Towel massage.* Rub your chest, stomach, hips, and thighs with a dry towel. Place it behind you, one end in each hand and saw back and forth, changing the vertical position from shoulders to buttocks. Do for just a few invigorating minutes.

The touch of another person is very important to us right from infancy. Scientists have discovered that a newborn child with eyes opened for the first time can differentiate between a mask and a human face. Children respond to cuddling and affection in very vital ways. Dwarfism, or retarded physical growth in a child, has been directly traced to a lack of this affection during early years.

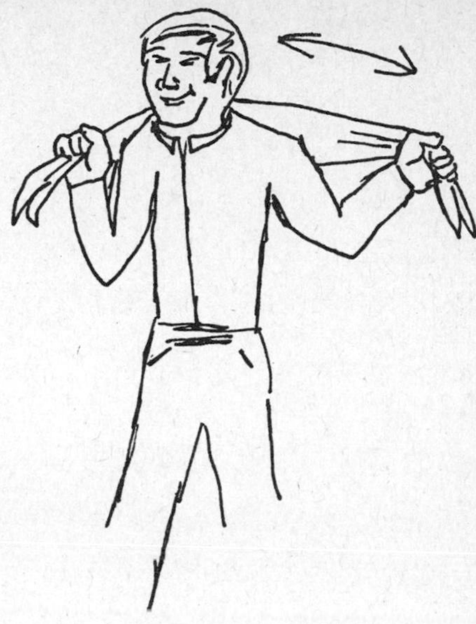

Figure 6-6

You can help another person to feel better by just showing you care. What better way than by giving that person a gentle:

- Neck rub
- Shoulder rub
- Back rub
- Foot rub

I use the word "gentle" because it translates into "safe." Don't get carried away with your own importance. Let your hands be loving as they move over the shoulder area. Move outwards from the center, and upwards, where neck and shoulders are being massaged. Here the person you are helping could be seated or standing.

The back massage requires a prone position. Move the fingers and palms up the upper spine, down the lower spine, and along the rib cage – gently.

The foot rub is a gentle kneading of the heel and arch. Then with one hand on the ankle, gently pull the foot, then each toe.

A five minute foot massage is a great way for two people to help each other to elevate their level of well-being.

One day we will understand better why some of these old practices work so well. Recently, scientists noted that a heart cell continues to beat or pulsate when removed from the body and placed in solution. Two such cells, from different people, will continue to beat at different rhythms. Then if the two cells happen to flow together and touch, they begin to beat in unison.

I am going to give you some specific ways to use your hands to help yourself with special problems in the chapters ahead, ways to apply pressure or to rub.

Hands have energy. Healers have been using the "laying on of hands" since Biblical days. So the massage is not only an old-fashioned remedy — it may be the first remedy.

7

OLD-FASHIONED REMEDIES THAT WORK WONDERS FOR STIFF NECKS AND TRICKY BACKS

Being in chiropractic I see so many people with horrible backaches that make walking difficult and painful. Many have filled their bodies with drugs that affect vital organs in order to relieve the pain, but to no avail.

Back pains seem to be the most persistent, as well as the most erratic. You may think it is gone, then you move in a certain way and that knife-like twinge hits you.

The steady pain is just as unbearable. It changes a blue sky to gray, making life hard to bear.

How can you read this chapter if you are in pain? So I am going to start this chapter with ways to relieve pain. These ways apply to pain in general, but back pains in particular.

DRUGLESS PAIN KILLERS THAT WORK BEST

Heat has been used in many ways to help pain. Perhaps the best known is the hot water bottle. A rubber container is filled with hot water, and it gives immediate relief to the pain of indigestion, rheumatism, and back problems.

Grandma used to heat up a stone in the stove or in the fireplace, wrap it up in a towel, and give it to Gramps to use in bed. Today, we have the electric pad as successor to the hot water bottle, and the heat lamp.

Heat via a warm bath or shower is also pain relieving. A hot compress is useful for more localized pain. It stimulates the circulation of blood to the affected part, permitting nature to do the healing work.

The sun is nature's own source of heat and one of the best to chase away pain, if you live in a temperate climate. Exposing painful areas to just a few minutes of the healing rays makes a difference.

Pain due to inflammation or infection near the skin surface can be relieved with a poultice of natural herbs. Slippery elm is an old favorite, so are mustard and corn meal, today a bit easier to obtain. Often, just plain local mud or clay will make an effective poultice. Wrapped in gauze and placed on the affected part, the minerals seem to work a natural improvement.

Water is another pain reliever. Warm springs become health spas wherever they appear. Cold water works better than hot for some people. A cold compress around the neck can work wonders for that painful crick. An ice compress numbs whatever joint or other part of the body it is placed in contact with.

Massage is also a pain reliever. The simple movement of hands over the back, shoulder, and limbs as described in the previous chapter, can be a big help to the person in pain. The distress of an overstuffed stomach is also relieved by a gentle massage in the abdomen area.

Pressure on certain parts of the body can relieve pain. Try this on your next headache: press gently on both temples (one or two inches to the side of your eyes) for about thirty seconds. Just where to press for what pain is too large a subject to cover in this book. It is similar to the needle points of acupuncture and is frequently known as Western acupuncture. Tried and true.

Oxygen is a pain reliever. This is especially effective when the pain has been caused by the lack of fresh air. Toxic conditions often result from stuffy rooms. Subways, exhaust-filled streets, smoky rooms, poison the body and the body cries out for oxygen by the only way it knows — pain. You don't need an oxygen mask attached to an oxygen tank. All you need is a few deep breaths of pure, clean, fresh air.

In the old days they liked to go out in the cool of a shade tree to fill their lungs. Their intuition was leading them correctly, because there is more oxygen where there is greenery. Green plants take in the carbon dioxide we exhale and release oxygen back into the atmosphere.

There are mental ways, too, of relieving pain. "Take your mind off it" goes the saying. What is meant is that the mind cannot be conscious of two things at the same time. If you are figuring out your next checker move, you cannot possibly feel the pain of your headache. The pain is still there, as you discover when the move is made, but meanwhile you have not been feeling that pain. And that's what counts.

If you can think of something else so absorbing that your thoughts stay with it — no pain.

Some people knew of self-hypnosis and positive thinking in those days, too. The story of Desmen had spread and so had the pain-killing properties of self-induced trances used by Indian Fakirs who could lie "painlessly" on a bed of nails. Then in the past century the power of the mind over the body was professionalized by Freud and popularized by Coué, who had thousands helping pain and other problems by looking in the mirror and repeating over and over again "Every day, in every way, I am getting better and better."

Today, more direct methods are used. You relax and, say the pain is in your wrist, you hang your hand in an imaginary bucket of ice water, "feeling" it get more and more numb. When you extract it mentally, the pain is gone.

You can use this for other parts of our body by going through the same procedure. Then touching the painful area with your numb hand, ordering the numbness to be transferred. And so it is.

Pain is nature's distress signal. It is usually indicative of abnormality. To remove pain is to turn off a warning light without checking out the possibilities. What I am really saying is: if the pain persists see your doctor.

THE COST OF CHEMICAL PAIN RELIEVERS

Water — hot or cold — is relatively free. So is the sunlight, oxygen-filled fresh air, a relative's friendly massage, and the other time-tested pain-killers I have suggested.

Aspirin is relatively free, too. The cost of a dose is measured in pennies, a small price to pay for headache relief or relief from the pain of arthritis.

But there is a far greater price to be paid after you take the dose. If you are a thrifty shopper like your grandfolks were, you will want to know the whole cost.

Aspirin is salicylic acid, Gleason's *Clinical Toxicology of Commercial Products, 4th Ed.* says that average doses, but more commonly large doses, can cause ringing in the ears, nausea, vomiting, diarrhea, and intestinal bleeding.

What about large doses? Acidosis, blurring of vision, rapid heart beat, hallucinations, and — in progressive order — convulsions, circulatory collapse, coma, respiratory failure, death.

What is a large dose? One teaspoonful which is estimated at twelve tablets. Now nobody in his right mind takes that many aspirin. But how about two or three, then another two or three, again and again? Twelve in a period of as many hours? That is skirting death fairly close.

Merck's Index, the guidebook of the pharmacy profession, says that prolonged use of average or large doses may inhibit blood clotting and result in hemorrhaging. It says also that large doses of aspirin usually used in cases of rheumatic fever can cause Cushing's syndrome which include such symptoms as curvature of the spine.

It seems ironic that one of the most widely used chemical pain killers itself produces a condition that is one of the most common causes of pain, — the back problem.

Would you prefer to buy another chemical pain-killer that is less risky than aspirin? Aspirin is an ingredient of many other pain-killing products. Even if it is not, there is no pain-killer that can be called harmless.

Maybe you will continue to take these chemical pain-killers. But at least now you know more about the price you pay.

Chemicals have their value. But Americans rely too heavily on them. With our affluence and technology you would think we would be the healthiest people in the world. It may come as a surprise to you that our death rate exceeds quite a few countries. In fact, we are so far down the list that you might call us among the unhealthiest. I do not have the very latest figures but those I do have, obtained from the United Nations, show that there are over eighty nations with a lower death rate than ours, — like Hong Kong, Israel, Iran, Syria, Cuba, even Viet Nam.

How do we compare with the Soviet Union? Their death rate is 7.1% compared to our 9.5%. Did you know that the Russians do not permit chemical additives to be put into their foods? The canning process is done by heat alone, the preserving process by sugar or freezing. The thousands of chemical additives used in American food technology are shunned by the Russians, as are tons of other chemicals we live, and die, by.

Nature, I hear you calling.

WHAT TO DO FOR A STIFF NECK

Well, so much for the relief of pain. Let's get to the cause now and see what we can do about that. And let's start with the neck and work down to the lower back.

John D., was a painting contractor. He came to me with a stiff, sore neck and headaches. He complained that his neck always seemed stiff and sore. Sometimes he got the headaches after painting overhead, such as ceilings and underneath house eaves, but they could come at other times, too.

He was given regular treatments at my office with instructions to do an easy neck motion. Within a week to ten days his neck was fine. He was discharged symptom free and pain free.

A year later I happened to meet John on the street one day. He told me he had had no real trouble with the stiff neck. However, he did say that whenever there was any slight stiffness in his neck, he would do the "Dr. Schneider Neck Exercise."

Now I don't lay claim to inventing the exercise. Its origins are lost in antiquity. But here is how it goes:

1. While standing, let the head move slowly forward and downward without forcing it.

2. Firmly interlace the fingers behind the neck.
3. Slowly bring the head upward as if to look at the ceiling directly above. Hold the head in this position for approximately thirty seconds.
4. Relax to normal position, resting two or three minutes.
5. Repeat the same procedure six times, starting with step 1 and resting after each stretching.

You can use this exercise effectively when the muscular stiffness and neck soreness is caused by exposure to cold air or wind and rain, excessive use, and even in some cases of whiplash.

There is an expression that has been around several generations: "That person gives me a pain in the neck." Your stiff neck may not be due to painting under eaves or "rubber-necking" on a sightseeing bus. It might very well be due to a mental stress that in turn causes a physical stress.

If anybody has been giving you difficulty just prior to the neck stiffness, that situation is suspect as the cause.

The cure? Insulate yourself emotionally — physically, too, with distance between you if circumstances permit — by adjusting to the situation. It is easier to say this than it is to do, but the mastering of one part tolerance, two parts understanding might be just the recipe your neck needs.

Earlier I mentioned wintergreen as an effective herb that is still a widely used remedy.

Have your druggist mix a solution of 15 percent oil of wintergreen and 85 percent rubbing alcohol. Apply this solution to the sore or stiff muscle area. (Be careful to keep this solution away from your eyes, mucous membranes, and do not take internally.) Rub very lightly. After the area is well coated, cover it with a hot damp cloth.

After applying, you will notice a mild dark redness of the skin. Although it will feel very hot, don't worry. It won't burn the normal skin. It is only a temporary condition for the skin. The reason for this redness is the combined action of the heat and the wintergreen-alcohol preparation which brings more blood to the surface of the skin, increasing circulation to the area that needs it.

This treatment has proven to be especially effective in the cases of stiff, sore neck problems that often develop into headaches or numbness of the hands and arms.

J. S., a salesman who drove several hundred miles each week, complained of a very stiff neck suffered while traveling in his territory. I treated him on weekends when he would return to his home town. The treatment would relieve the stiffness until he was back on the road. I recommended he use this wintergreen and rubbing alcohol solution in the evenings before retiring. The next weekend he returned to my office telling me how much better his neck and shoulders were feeling.

HOW TO PREVENT BACKACHE FROM CREEPING UP ON YOU WHILE YOU ARE ASLEEP

Numerous cases on record show that backache, particularly in the lumbo-sacral (lower back) area, as well as pain in the neck and shoulders, has been arrested by the simple act of changing the habitual sleeping position.

One such case is J. L., secretary, who had suffered with recurring headaches over a period of three years. Upon examination of her cervical spine (neck), several vertebrae were found to be rotated (turned).

I questioned her about her sleeping position. She stated she usually slept on her "tummy," which I believe was causing the distortion in her neck and her headaches. She was instructed not to go to sleep on her abdomen, but to assume a position on her back or side. Both knees should be bent and drawn up together approximately one-half way.

I explained to her that this position would help alleviate any possibility of soreness and stiffness in the lower back by allowing a more relaxed position of the spinal column.

She was also instructed to use a smaller pillow than she had been using and to position the pillow closer to under her neck, with less elevation under the head than under her neck.

Within ten days of treatments for the distortion and ten nights of her following the instructions for changing her sleeping position, her headaches were completely relieved, and of course, she was resting much easier.

Another recommendation I have given countless people to aid their rest and sleep is the use of a bed board.

An inexpensive sheet of ½ inch thick plywood cut the full size (length and width) of the mattress and placed between mattress and springs can do a lot to firm up a too soft, "rolling" mattress. Many backaches and tiredness have been greatly helped by adding this rigidity to mattress and spring.

"A soft mattress is hard on your back," agrees a voice from the past.

WHAT YOU CAN DO AT HOME TO PREVENT BACK TROUBLE

Back problems are on the increase because we are getting further and further away from nature in our life style.

We sleep on tricky mattresses and so invite tricky backs.

We push harder than we should, forgetting "tomorrow is another day."

We work in artificial environments and in unnaturally cramped positions, or we sit on a chair at a desk that creates its own back position and ignores ours.

I believe I should sleep on a firm mattress.

I believe I should stretch in the morning to loosen up my muscles.

I believe I should be conscious of my posture standing and walking, seeking to be erect.

I believe that I should not overdo physical effort — recognizing and starting within my limits.

I believe in getting help to lift heavy objects.

I believe my legs need to bend and do their share, rather than making my back do all the bending.

I believe that when I must do desk work or work in a cramped position that I get up at frequent intervals and give those cramped muscles a chance to "breathe."

I believe in keeping my spine in balance and avoiding sudden bending, twisting, or jerking.

Now I believe all this and I try to practice this, but I did not learn it in chiropractic. Maybe its study refreshed my memory, but somehow I already accepted this as common sense — maybe I learned it from my parents, or my grandparents.

It pays to take good care of your back. This I did learn in chiropractic. I have seen how spinal pressure can cause tension on nerves by robbing vital organs of essential nerve energy.

A back problem may not manifest as a back pain or twinge. Such symptoms as headaches, painful joints, pain between the shoulders, or numbness in arms, hands, or legs can be a result of a back that needs care and attention.

HOME REMEDIES FOR THE ACHING BACK

This is going to be a short section of this chapter. Home remedies for the aching back? Very few. I have already told you how to relieve the pain. I have made suggestions to prevent back trouble. But once that trouble arrives, there is little short of professional care that will help.

You hear a lot about exercise to cure common back pain. But if I were to tell you on these pages to move your aching back through all kinds of paces you would have good reason to think mighty unkindly of me.

How can you even think of exercise when you are in pain. Every sudden motion is a risk of stabbing twinge.

Some 95% of common back pains are due to structural disrelations in the spine. These cause interference with nerve functioning. Sometimes a nerve is actually pinched. Exercise can only irritate the situation.

However, "movements" and "exercises" are two different kettles of fish. I am going to give you some slow, easy movements to perform which will make your back feel good.

The professional chiropractors are trained to deal with back problems. You might say it is one of their specialties. A ten year study of back pain cases in the Workmen's Compensation files spanning five states showed that, under medical care, back patients lost an average of thirty-three days from work, while under chiropractic care the average lost time from work was one week.

Once you see your health care specialist, then home exercise may be prescribed. He may recommend isometric exercises where you contract your muscles forcibly for a few moments, like standing with one shoulder against the inside of a door frame and pushing with the other hand against the opposite side of the frame; or pushing the head with the palms of the hand, sideways, forwards, or back. Your doctor will prescribe the right motions for your condition and give you the amount of time to hold these muscle-forcing positions.

I am going to suggest a few exercises for special back conditions on one condition: that if you are under the care of a doctor, you get his permission before you begin doing these movements.

A HOME REMEDY FOR "SWAY BACK"

A condition known as "sway back" has been around for a long time. It has been understood to be a weakness of the muscles on either side of the spine on the back side of the abdominal cavity. This causes a swaying forward of the back.

If you try to strengthen these muscles, you can lessen the abnormal amount of curve in the lower back or lumbo-sacral area. You can also firm and flatten the abdomen.

Here is how it goes *(Figure 7-1):*

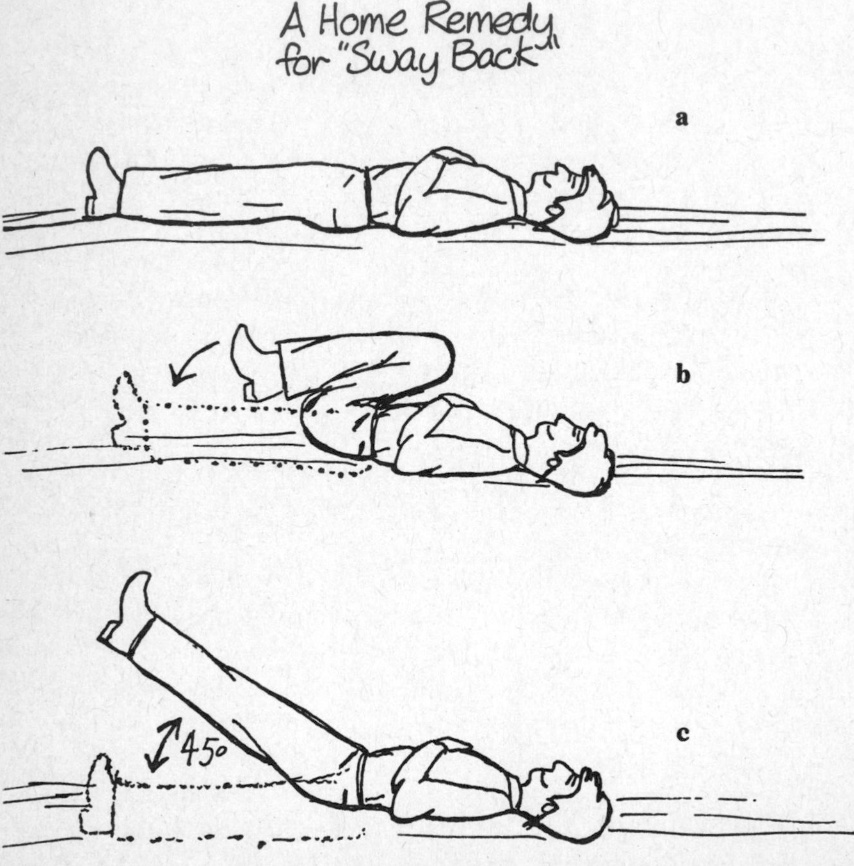

Figure 7-1

A Home Remedy for "Sway Back"

1. Lie flat on your back on the floor.
2. Bending the knees, bring them together to the abdomen.
3. Straighten out the legs, laying them once again flat on the floor.
4. Now holding both legs straight and rigid, and by bend-at the hips, pull both legs up to an approximate forty-five degree angle with the floor. Care should be taken not to rapidly jerk the legs upward so as to not strain the abdominal muscles.
5. Slowly lower the legs (keeping them rigid) to the floor.

The number of times you repeat this exercise is up to your discretion. I recommend a gradual increase in the number of times that you raise and lower the legs each day.

Frank B. had had a chronic low back pain for fifteen years. He had consulted several doctors. Some had given him temporary relief, but the old problem would always return. I treated Frank for a period of two weeks. I recommended he do this exercise in the morning before arising and again when first retiring at night, a half dozen times each session. He responded very rapidly and was discharged with no more pain at the end of two weeks.

Two years later I happened to meet Frank at a luncheon, and he was telling me how wonderful he felt since the last time I had seen him professionally. He said he had been doing his exercises faithfully even if his back was not bothering him. I was very happy to hear his comments, because it confirmed what I have tried to teach so many of my patients, namely that this exercise is also a preventive measure, especially since it maintains a normal flexion of the muscles of the lower spine.

If you have had surgery, or if you are under a doctor's care, check with your surgeon or doctor before doing this exercise, or for that matter, any other exercise.

CORRECTIVE MOVEMENTS YOU CAN DO FOR LOWER BACKACHE

Here is another movement sequence that releases and relaxes. Again, if you are in treatment or considering it, consult your health care specialist before going through these movements.

These movements are done while lying flat on the floor. They help the muscles throughout the lower lumbar area of the spine. Here are the steps to take *(Figure 7-2).*

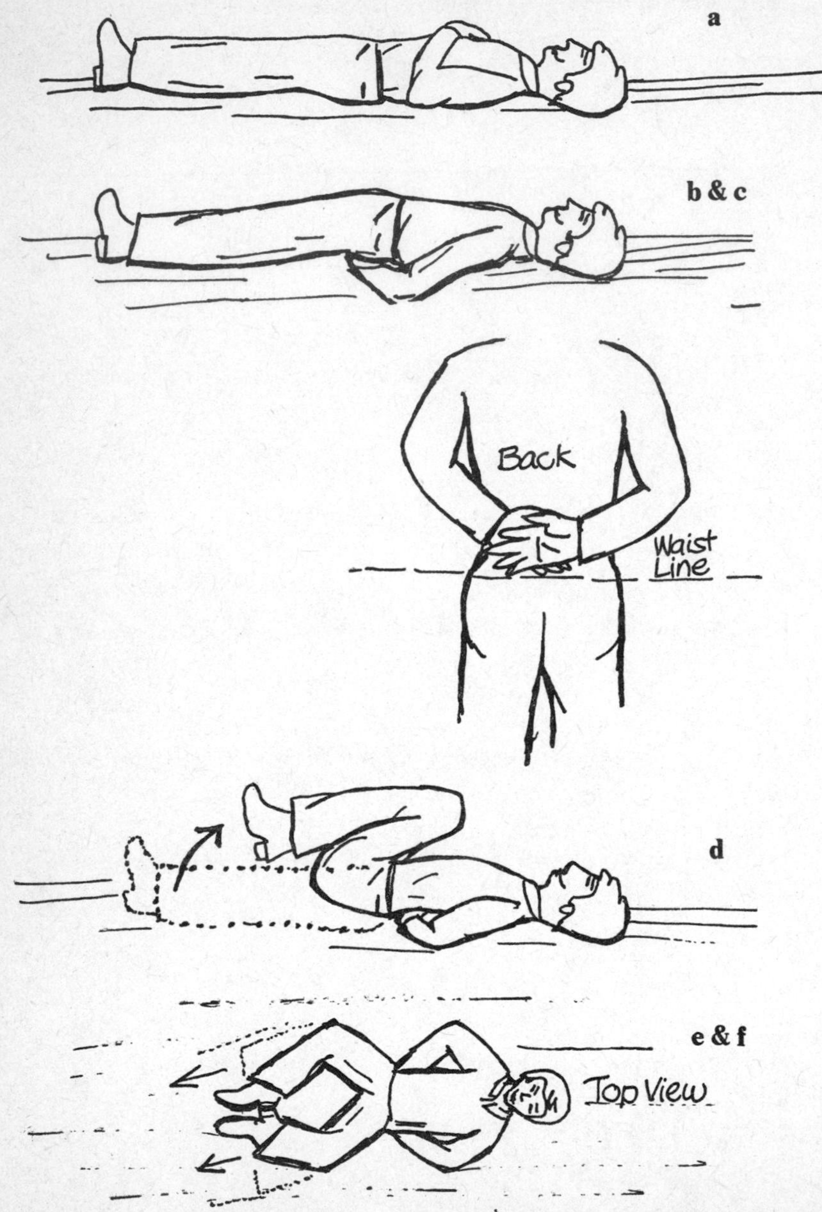
Corrective Movements
You Can Do For Lower Back Ache
a
b & c
Back
Waist
Line
d
e & f
Top View

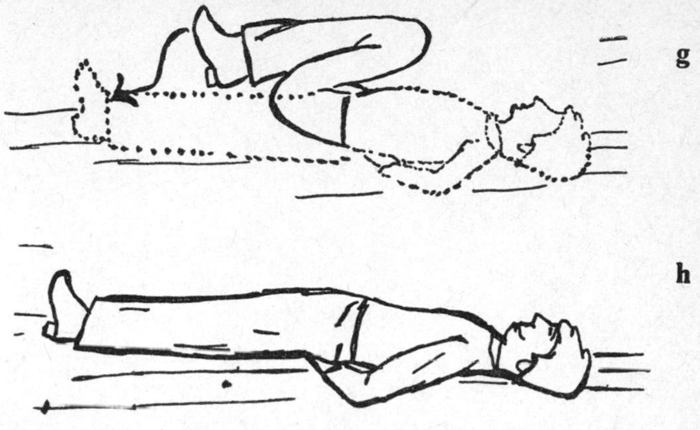

Figure 7-2

a. Lie flat on the back, perferably on a firm surface such as the floor.
b. Raise the hips off the floor two inches.
c. Place one hand upon the other (flat) behind you under the hips so that the top edge of the hands will be approximately in line with the waistline.
d. Lie upon your hands, raising both legs with knees bent toward the abdomen.
e. Spread the knees as far apart as possible, keeping the feet touching. Do not let the feet touch the floor.
f. Straighten out the legs feetward.
g. Let the feet relax to the floor after the legs have been extended.
h. Lie quietly for five minutes.

You may hear a snapping sound, especially if you have gone through these movements properly. Do not be alarmed as this merely indicates a relaxing of the muscles involved.

Of all the basic movements for back trouble handed down by word of mouth or adopted by health care training institutions, this one I have found to be the most successful. In my 25 years of practice, every patient that faithfully performed these motions had virtually no more problems with his back, and some I have seen ten years later and this is still true. With one exception: Mr. H. returned after nine years with a back problem. But he had just slipped and fallen while unloading a bag of cement from his truck.

Here is another position you can get yourself into that helps lower-back distress. It gives good flexion to the spinal discs and stretches the lower-back muscles.

Grandma G. was a nimble little lady in her seventies. She had always believed in exercising and eating good healthy foods. Grandma had been working in her garden one day and apparently "overdid" her lower back while pulling and hoeing weeds. She came to me in a very bent-over-forward position. She was truly in misery. After examination and treatment she was instructed to do this knee-chest exercise that evening before retiring and again the following morning. The next day I saw her again. She was very happy with this motion that I had taught her to do. It's really quite simple:

a. Assume a kneeling (not squatting) position, making sure the buttocks are resting on the heels.
b. Bend forward letting the chest touch the knees.
c. Crawl forward so that the thighs are at a ninety-degree angle with the floor.
d. Move the buttocks back to the original starting position.
e. Repeat this exercise six to eight times morning or evening, as your doctor recommends.

There is an exercise wheel that is sold in most sporting-goods stores. It permits a movement very similar to the one I have just described *(Figure 7-3).*

Mrs. C., in her forties, had a chronic complaint of soreness in her lower back. She also complained that it took her one half of the morning just to wake up and think straight. I suggested an exercise much likened to a cat's stretch. The recommendation was to purchase the wheel and to use it each morning upon first arising. She was to do this by kneeling on the floor and pushing (rolling) the wheel back and forth across the floor twelve times, increasing by two times each morning until she was rolling it thirty-six times.

a
b
c & d
90°
The same
movements except
with the wheel

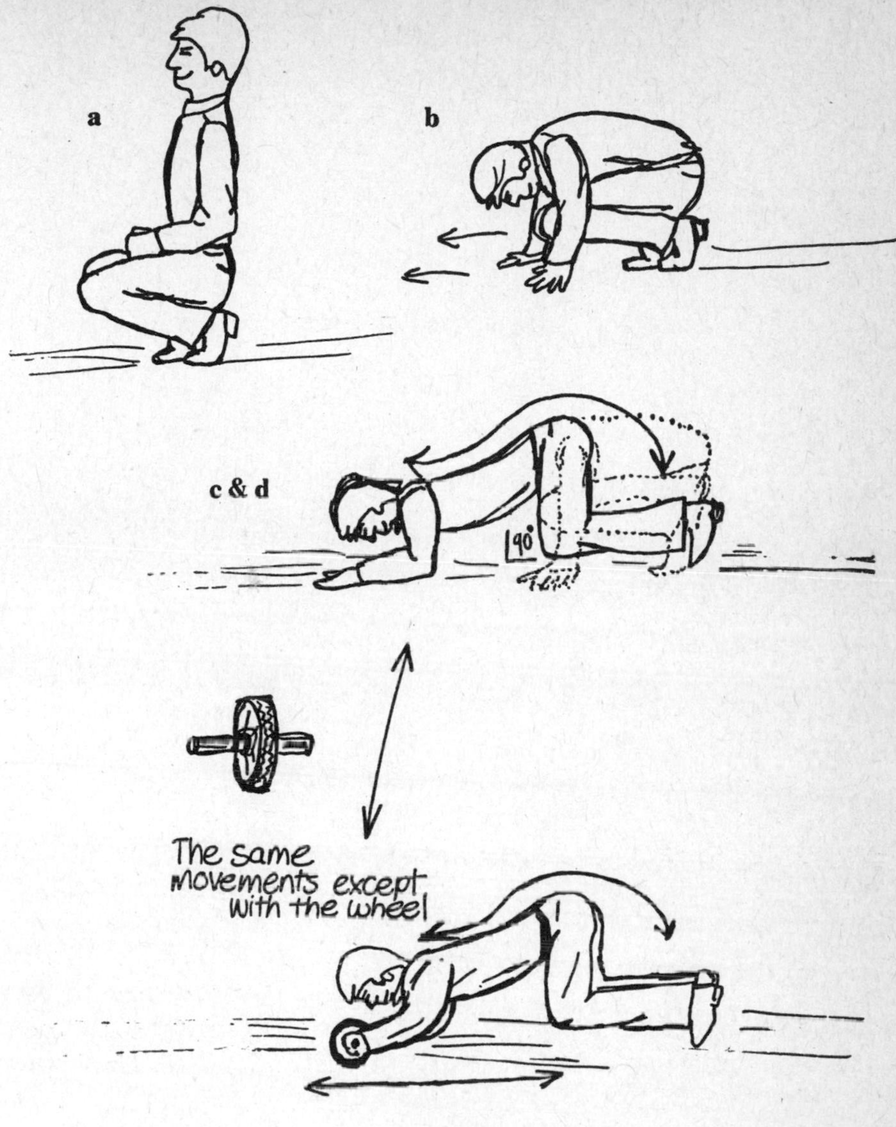

Figure 7-3

This simple series of movements took no more than three to five minutes per day. A week later she returned to my office telling me of the wonderful wide-awake feeling she now had. She said she could think much more clearly early in the morning. She also felt that it had helped eliminate the soreness in her lower back.

THE TRUTH ABOUT YOUR BACK TROUBLE

About six in the morning a doctor's phone rings. The lady on the other end of the line is quite excited.

"Doctor, just now my husband bent over to tie his shoe and he can't straighten up. I helped him down on the bed. He won't move."

"Where is the pain?" the doctor asks.

"He said a catch struck him in the back and then traveled right down to his hip. Now, he says, the pain goes all the way down to his calf."

"Put hot towels on his back for fifteen minutes, then get some help and get him into the office. Phone me when you leave and I'll be waiting for you when you arrive."

The doctor takes X-rays when the patient arrives and finds misplacements of the fourth and fifth lumbar vetebrae — the two lowest spinal joints. He gives the man an adjustment and the man is able to walk out under his own power.

Now the reason I tell you this story is that while getting a case history on this patient, the doctor finds that he had experienced mild episodes of this lower-back pain over the past four or five years. In other words, it did not just strike like lightning out of the blue. It had been brewing and sending its warning signals, but these warnings had been largely ignored.

Back problems have been the toughest to cure at home. The old folks talked about "my sciatica" as if those back, hip, and leg pains were here to stay. Without professional help, chances are they were right.

If you get early warning signals about your back, heed them. Make a change in the way you walk, sit, work, play and sleep, using the preventive suggestions that are at the beginning of this chapter.

8

WHAT TO DO ABOUT FRAZZLED NERVES, THE SHAKES, AND JUMPINESS

"I've got jittery nerves."

"She's irritable."

"He's got a short temper."

More and more people are complaining about frazzled nerves, fidgity fingers, jumpiness, and the shakes. Some say it is due to our faster pace; others say it is due to the population explosion and resulting crowding. Still others point to our mineral depleted food.

Let's say all three reasons are valid. What, then, do we do about it?

Nerves are literally vital to life. They control all vital organs. They transmit all sensory input to the brain — sight, sound, touch, taste, and smell. Nerves maintain your sense of balance, keep your body temperature near 98.6°, permit you to swallow, control your blood pressure, control your heart, regulate your digestive organs, move your bowels, and regulate your respiration.

Nervousness can derive from outside causes or inside causes.

Outside causes are excessive noise levels around you, too much activity, pressure of time, moods and excitement of other people, irritation from unwanted circumstances or from exasperating people, loneliness, lack of sexual satisfaction, and just plain worry or anxiety.

These are usually prolonged situations that last long enough to produce wear and tear on the nerves.

Internal causes can come from a lack of nourishment for the nerves or a physical impairment, such as pinching of certain nerves.

Of course, the latter kind of internal cause needs the help of a professional health care practitioner. The doctor of chiropractic was one of the first to recognize that internal obstructions to the nerves must be removed in order for the body to function in its natural state of good health. He knows how to analyze and test the spine and nervous system to locate the cause of nervousness and nerve malfunction, and then to correct blocked or pinched nerves.

One of the places he will be examining for jittery nerves will be the neck area. A nerve difficulty near the top of the spine can cause nervous prostration. At the very top of the spine, where it joins the skull, are the nerves that, when pinched, can cause dizziness, insomnia, headache, and general nervousness.

But there are many natural remedies available to help your jittery nerves when such internal causes are not involved. Our grandparents knew what foods to take that were "good for the nerves" and how to compensate for outside causes of inner commotion.

HOW TO CONTROL YOUR NERVES BY YOUR OUTLOOK

Ever see two people confronted with the same situation? The first is wringing his hands with worry, the second wringing his hands about the first wringing his hands.

The worriers frazzle their own nerves. They also get on the nerves of the non-worriers.

I can sit here until doomsday telling you not to worry and it would not be worth a hoot to you. But maybe there are a few things I can tell you that your non-worrying, philosophical forebears knew and which maybe you need to be reminded of. I am going to do this first and then hand out some natural remedies later.

First, do you know that the world does not have you by the tail? You have the world by the tail. Some people can look at the same glass and see it half full, others see it half empty. Same world, same glass, different outlooks.

Now, I would get all nervous and fidgety if I could not convince you that you really had the world by the tail, instead of the way you think it is. I would become frustrated and, to use a modern expression, "up-tight."

So I let you be the way you want to be, and as a result I am better off myself. Nervousness hurts only the one who is nervous. When you get up a head of steam you're going to blow your own valve, nobody else's.

For your own selfish good, if you are the nervous type, you need to cultivate some new attitudes and outlooks. If you don't, all the remedies in the world laid end-to-end would not reach your rising gorge.

What attitudes? An attitude of:

- Thanks for what you have instead of bitterness over what you don't have.
- Self-acceptance, instead of taking what someone else says about you as the gospel truth.
- Patience, knowing the pot will boil if you'd only stop looking at it.
- Solutions, not problems. See the best happening, not the worst.
- Fun and good humor instead of fear.

In previous chapters I gave you mental exercises to do to help you relax and also physical things to do to help you relax. Here is a successful method to combine the two:

1. Sit in a comfortable chair.
2. Be aware of your toes and ankles. Wiggle your toes, move your ankles, get them loosened up.
3. Let your awareness move to your calves, legs, knees,

and thighs. Check out all the muscles. Ask them to relax.

4. Do the same for your hips, back, chest, and shoulders.
5. Let your arms hang limp by your sides or on your lap. Feel how relaxed they are. Talk to them.
6. Talk to your neck and shoulder muscles: "Relax, muscles."
7. Check your mouth and jaw. Feel comfortable in these areas. No tension.
8. Feel the liquid comfort of your eyes.
9. Smooth the brow.
10. Check out the little muscles of the scalp.

You are now relaxed from head to toe. It is a good feeling. All the cells of your body love it.

A COMMON HOUSEHOLD ITEM THAT RELIEVES SOME OF THE HARMFUL EFFECTS OF TENSION

The old folks knew that when pressure is used on nerve endings, it has a relaxing effect on the entire body.

The simple way of using this method is to clip five regular spring-type clothespins over the tip (one-half inch) of each finger of one hand including the thumb. Leave these clothespins in place for five to ten minutes. Then remove them and place them on the thumb and finger tips of the other hand in the same way. Do this after the evening meal or during the day if you feel it necessary. *(Figure 8-1)*

This therapy may sound rather foolish, but it does work.

Mrs. Joy S. came to my office with pain and numbness in her left arm. She explained to me that several years before she had had a serious injury to the arm. For two weeks prior to coming to me she had noticed the arm going to sleep, numbness, loss of strength in her hand, and at times a tingling feeling in her fingers. She told me at the beginning of the consultation that because of their limited income only one treatment would have to correct the condition.

I recommended that Mrs. S. put spring-type clothespins on the ends of each finger and thumb for five minutes each in the morning and in the evening. She thought this rather amusing, but agreed she would try anything.

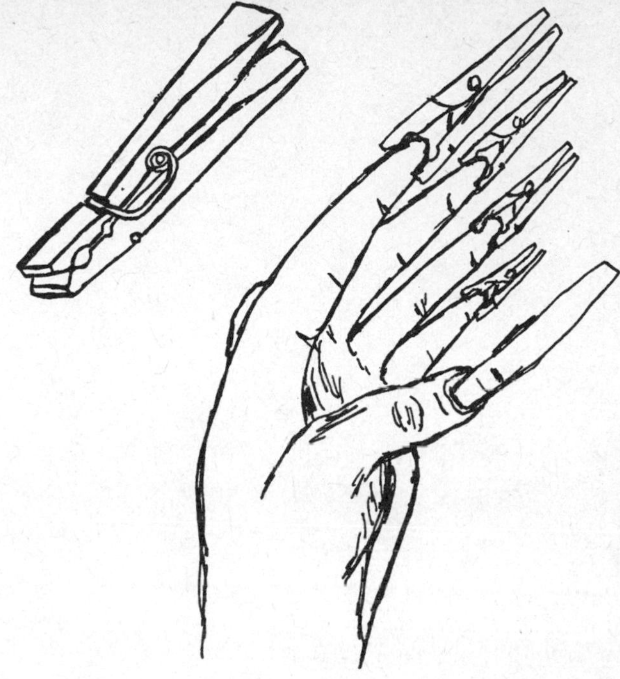

Figure 8-1

I asked her to phone within two weeks after starting this home therapy to let me know the results. She called two weeks later and she was happy to report in her estimation "ninety percent of the pain" had been alleviated.

HOW TO RELIEVE NERVOUSNESS RESULTING FROM WORRY OR EXCITEMENT

Grandma is brewing some valerian tea. That means Gramps must be on the war path. And if he is really tense and excited about something, she will probably add some celery seed, rosemary, and lemon.

Just the way coffee and tea are instant stimulators, herb teas can be instant relaxers. Tea made of the valerian root seems to have been the one most relied upon in the old days.

There are other natural sedatives in common herbs and foods. Take the old reliable apple. Some old folks swore it was the best nerve tonic, especially when juiced and taken on an empty stomach before retiring.

Vegetables that are said to be good for the nerves include artichoke, avocado, Brussels sprouts, cauliflower, and lettuce. Fruits that soothe the nerves are said to include papaya and the white grape.

On the other hand, sugar is said to induce a number of nervous afflictions.

The chemistry involved in feeding the nerves is a complicated matter. Any meal with a large amount of sugar and starch draws upon the body's store of thiamine (vitamin B1). If there is not enough thiamine available, these starches are insufficiently digested forming two acids: lactic and pyruvic. These acids irritate the nerves. When thiamine, or B1, is taken the person feels more relaxed and less ready to fly off the handle.

Nerves require constant nourishment and without it degenerate at a more rapid rate than other tissues.

Their chief needs are calcium, magnesium, thiamine, and glutamic acid. The calcium and magnesium seem to be essential in the nerve ability to transmit or telegraph messages to the brain. The thiamine and glutamic acid appear to help the brain cells to communicate through the nerves.

Grains have a good percentage of nerve food — not refined grain, but whole grain. Peanuts are good, and almonds. So are raisins. Combine all of these with whole wheat and you have a splendid breakfast cereal that will help you start the day with a pleasant disposition.

When calcium levels are low in the blood supply, the person feels an inability to relax. Sleep is difficult. There is irritability. If the calcium lack is critical, muscle cramps or spasms can result, usually in the legs or feet.

Since menstruation saps the calcium supply, many women experience nervousness and even depression during the days preceding and during menstrual flow.

A good source of calcium is milk and the old faithful cure for restlessness at night — a glass of warm milk — is still popular today. I do not advocate the use of cow's milk. Goat's milk is superior. Magnesium is a component of chlorophyll, so it is found in all leafy green vegetables.

Because of their content of these nerve nutrients, the following foods are good care for nervousness:

- Tomatoes
- Carrots
- Turnips
- Leafy green vegetables
- Kidney beans
- Dry beans
- Soy beans
- Lentils
- Fish
- Whole grains
- Nuts
- Pork
- Lemon juice (glutamic acid)

Sometimes nervousness is the result of a toxic condition in the body. Anything in nature's storehouse that cleanses the body of accumulated poisons thus becomes an acid in such cases. That is why apples come back into the picture, not just the juice, but now the whole apple. The apple rind contains pectin which helps to clear noxious substances from the body and also retards the spoiling of protein matter in the intestines.

Camomile is available in tea form in specialty food shops. Its name comes from the Greek meaning "ground apple," as its odor is somewhat like that of an apple. Its affect on the nerves is just as soothing as an apple. The tea is prepared from the flowers and is also good for indigestion. Camomile goes way back to early Colonial days and even further. It is said to have been used by the Egyptians to prevent aging.

NERVOUS DISORDERS THAT BEAR WATCHING

Little frustrations can grow to huge threats. A person who ignores his own ugly moods is accepting them as a way of life.

We doctors often get patients with serious physical disorders that we can trace to mental problems. These mental problems in turn started with nervousness, tension, and irritability.

An apple or camomile tea is not going to do anything for the woman who is worried day-in and night-out that her husband is seeing another woman.

A glass of warm milk may help a business man go to sleep, but when he awakens once again to the problem of employees, or cash flow, or sagging sales, that tension is back again doing its dirty work.

You can treat the symptom as a temporary measure, but pretty soon you are going to have to get to the root of the problem.

Here is a typical case that has gone too long.

A woman comes to the office. I ask her the nature of her problem. Suddenly she bursts into tears.

"Doctor something is happening to me. I scream at the children, shout at my husband. Everything annoys me. I am constantly afraid — I don't know of what — like there is tragedy just around the corner."

She cries some more, then continues.

"I have not had a good night's sleep in months. Doctor, is it possible I am going out of my mind?"

Of course it is possible. Indeed probable. But I don't tell her so. She is headed for a nervous breakdown and they come in all shapes and sizes. Thing is, she can begin an improvement immediately.

If she can afford to go to a psychologist or a psychiatrist, this kind of professional help can identify the basic problem and lend help in handling it. This is a relatively new approach, unknown to most people a century ago.

What did they do a century ago? Either they took a long trip or they quit running and they turned and faced up to the problem.

Today we run. We run from doctor to doctor and from sedation to sedation. There must be ten million Americans on tranquilizers and other nerve sedatives today. This is an attempt to escape. But there really is no escape on this route.

The standard prescription in the old days was "take a vacation." The bigger the problem and the richer the patient, the longer the trip. Some were advised to take a trip around the world. Today the world is smaller. It is harder to get away from anything or anybody.

Today we have no choice but to get in touch with our own feelings. When we do, we may find that the real cause is a question of

- Ego
- Pride
- Jealousy
- Unfounded fear

- Suspicion
- Unwarranted guilt

If allowed to fester, any of these personality imbalances can cause as much of a health problem as an infection. Maybe worse — there are no white blood corpuscles to come to our aid and in these situations we need to come to our own aid.

AN IMAGINARY MIRROR THAT CAN HELP YOU

Fortunately, there *is* an answer. It is not easy to come by, but the moment we just start approaching it we get relief. Nervousness recedes.

That answer lies in the word "self-image."

A person with a poor opinion of himself needs to build up his ego; has vulnerable pride; becomes easily jealous, afraid, and suspicious; and is plagued by guilt.

How do you change your self-image?

There are methods today based on the Coué method — "Every day in every way I am getting better and better." They are methods of reconditioning yourself away from all the put-downs that have limited your own opinion of yourself. They involve positive statements about yourself, positive images, positive reprogramming, but in a way that you can believe and accept.

These include the mind courses like Silva Mind Control, the skill courses like Dale Carnegie, and just plain study in philosophy and religion devoted to recognizing the divinity in yourself.

The key is getting to appreciate yourself. That is the opposite of depreciate, which others tend to do to us from classroom to grave.

Books on self-hypnotism* and auto-conditioning help, but you have to put these books down from time to time, stop reading, and start doing.

The inclination is not to do anything. You like to feel the way you do about yourself. That's the way you are.

But the price of not changing is exorbitant: A poor self-image leads to phobias and other nervous causes spelled out above. This nervousness can become aggravated and lead to:

---

*Sidney Petrie and Robert B. Stone, *Hypno-Cybernetics,* (West Nyack, N.Y.: Parker Publishing Co., 1974).

- An occasional vice-like pain around the rim of the skull
- Chronic headache
- Insomnia
- Twitching of the muscles
- Excessive perspiration
- Palpitations of the heart
- Hot flashes
- Dizziness
- Weakness and fatigue
- Shortness of breath or breathing difficulty
- Dryness of the mouth
- Constriction of the throat, difficulty in swallowing
- Tightness between shoulders, pain in chest
- Heartburn
- Excessive stomach gas, belching
- Constipation
- Diarrhea

Take your pick. One of them, two of them, all of them. And this is only the beginning. Each leads to others. Can you imagine where dizziness may lead to? Or palpitations? Or shortness of breath?

Then there are scores more symptoms I did not list, but one in particular:

- Hypochondria.

This is the ability of the imagination to dream up symptoms. *Question:* What's so bad about imagined health problems? *Answer:* They can come true. Graveyards are full of dead bodies, the victims of imagined illnesses that eventually killed them.

Had enough? I'm not one for scare psychology or I'd be causing exactly what I am trying to get you to cure.

But I want to motivate you to do something about your opinion of yourself. If you suffer from "nerves" — and if it is not caused by nutritional deficiency (see all the nerve foods at the beginning of this chapter) — you need to take another look at yourself.

This is what I meant by facing the problem squarely, instead of running away from it via the pillbox.

Now, maybe you do not want to take any course, or go to any clinic, or read any more books. So I am going to give you a simple way to change your appreciation of yourself, get rid of your unwanted pains and aches, and steady your nerves.

I'll tell you what to do then you put the book down and do it:

1. Look at yourself in the mirror.
2. Leave the mirror and relax in a chair.
3. Take a few minutes to quiet down even more.
4. Close your eyes and "see" yourself again as if you were looking in the mirror.
5. Expand the picture to include relatives, boss, office, – anything that may be at the root of "nerves."
6. Now erase the picture.
7. Substitute a new picture. See yourself as you want to be. More attractive, more appreciated and loved, more successful.
8. Say out aloud, "This begins to happen the moment I love myself."
9. Say to your image in this new picture, again out aloud, "I love you."

Now this is not necessarily exactly how the old folks cured nervousness resulting from the factors that I have pointed to, but these factors did not occur as frequently then as they do today.

The price of civilization can come high.

A final word about drugs. You may find it harder to say you love yourself or to confront your own emotions in a candid self-examination than to open an aspirin bottle. But remember that the aspirin is just delaying the moment of self-reckoning.

And if you delay too long...aspirins can cause internal bleeding and other pain killers, besides eventually damaging the brain, can meanwhile, according to Dr. Naphine A. Roe of Cornell University, interfere with the body's ability to absorb or properly utilize minerals and vitamins and possibly even replenish the body's own blood supply.

So you would be going in the opposite direction of our forefathers. They believed that health was a natural state — that it came from nature.

Be in touch with your own nature.

TIPS FOR WOMEN ONLY

I want to say a few words to the women so, men, skip this section.

You know how many women used to get themselves out of the dumps by going out and buying themselves a new hat or a new dress.

Now that may have not made the men folks feel any better when the ladies did this, but it can surely provide a lift to the feminine morale.

Any time a woman does something to make herself more beautiful and attractive she calms her nerves and builds up her self-image.

Then the beauty really begins to show because with calmer nerves, a woman radiates her true self.

Here is a program for a few hours devoted to *you.* I will list the possibilities; you put the program together to suit yourself.

1. Relax with a glass of nature's own nerve tonic — wine. Make it sherry. Sit in a comfortable chair, turn on some soft music (not rock), smell the bouquet of the wine and sip it slowly.
2. Let your mind daydream to its favorite subjects. How about a prince and princess type of fairy tale, just for starters?
3. Do something creative. Improve a dress with embroidery. Paint a picture. Write a poem. Move a few vases around. Arrange some flowers.
4. Take a warm bath, or shower, or sauna. If there is a masseuse available, make an appointment or give yourself a massage.
5. Give yourself a beauty treatment. Go to the beauty parlor or use face cream, hand lotion and other beauty aids leisurely and in ways that you never took the time to before.

6. Fix your hair in a new way or improve the old way.
7. Put on some daring make-up. A different color lipstick or eye shadow.
8. Give yourself a manicure or a pedicure or both.
9. Put on some dress or accessory that you usually save for a special occasion.
10. Take a walk. Feel nature's beauty. Feel your own beauty.

SIMPLE BODY PRESSURES THAT RELIEVE NERVOUS PRESSURE

Tension needs your special attention. Ignore it, suffer it, hope it will go away, and you are only inviting it to come home to roost. Its' nesting place can be your back, your stomach, your heart, your brain.

K. D., a middle-aged man, had a coronary a year before consulting me. Now he had at the time of my examination severe chest pains suggestive of angina. The treatment I gave relieved a certain amount of his discomfort.

I also instructed him to massage the web structure between the finger and the thumb of the left hand, applying hand cream for lubrication before beginning.

He was instructed to do a milking-pinching type of massage with the finger and thumb of the right hand, applying enough pressure to the web between the finger and thumb of the left hand to make it hurt. When I demonstrated, he really winced. This massaging was to be practiced for five minutes daily *(Figure 8-2)*.

One week later he returned to my office greatly relieved of the chest pain. I put pressure on the web of his left hand. No wince this time. In fact, there was very little discomfort to him. Apparently, he had been using this massage quite regularly. The more this is massaged, the more the tenderness in the hand and chest will disappear. I have recommended this technique for a great number of shoulder and chest conditions and have seen it work wonders in the majority of cases, especially those with prolonged tension as the original cause.

There are many nerve endings in the hands in the webbing or structure between thumb and finger, the thumbs, fingers, and in the palm of the hand.

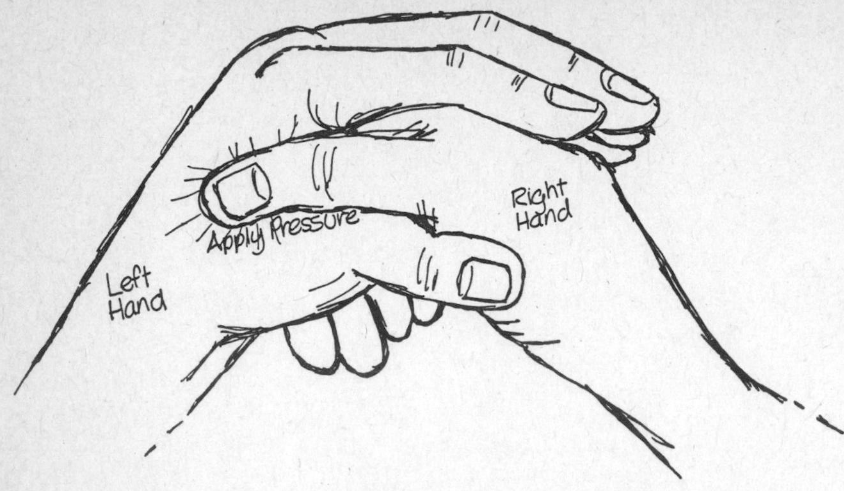

Figure 8-2

Milking-Pinching Type Finger Thumb Massage

Apply a hand lotion to these areas. Then massage or goad them with the fingers or thumb of the opposite hand for a period of five minutes twice a day or until the tension is relieved.

The pioneer women seemed to have an intuitive wisdom about rubbing in places that had no apparent bearing on the problem to the logical thinking of the pioneer men. It was as if they knew about acupuncture being used on the other side of the world.

"Jennie, it's not my hands, its my chest."

"Be still. You'll see."

And he usually did.

Another rub was used which I still have my patients do with good results.

I call it the shoulder release for deeper breathing. Nervous people frequently breathe shallowly. Often this is due to tension in the muscle structure which forms the shoulder girdle. You can release the shoulders to permit deeper natural breathing by this simple pressure *(Figure 8-3):*

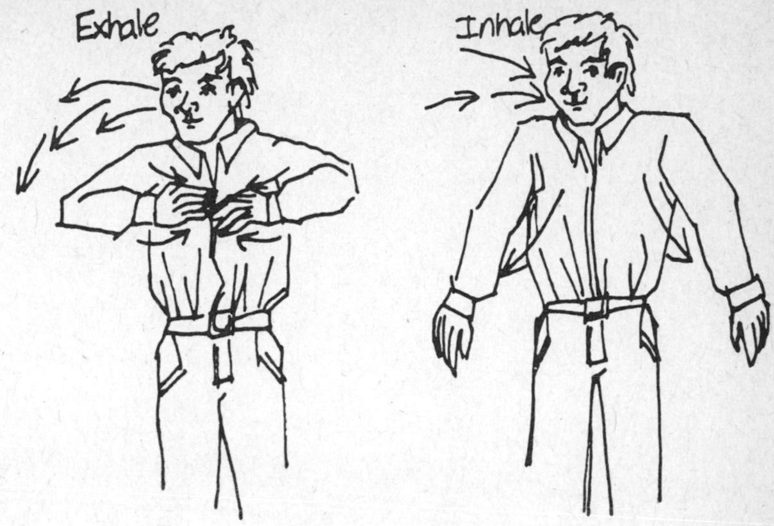

Figure 8-3

Shoulder Release for Deeper Breathing

1. While standing, place both hands high on the rib cage as near the armpits as possible.
2. Press inward as far as possible with both hands at the same time, exhaling through the open mouth.
3. Suddenly release both hands at the same time.
4. Inhale deeply, holding the breath for five seconds.

Repeat this exercise three to six times, which is usually sufficient to create a relaxation.

One of the most strength-sapping symptoms of anxiety, tension, frazzled nerves, and the jitters is loss of sleep.

Insomnia plagues millions of people in today's civilized world. Years ago, folks could doze off at the drop of a straw hat.

Since sleep is so important to our health — natural sleep — I am devoting the next chapter entirely to this subject.

9

HOW TO TURN RESTLESS NIGHTS INTO SOLID SLEEP

In the old days, cellars were entered from hatch doors on the side of the house. They would squeak when you opened them because the hinges were exposed to the elements and rusted easily.

When you opened these doors in the middle of the day, a draft of cold air would hit you. This was the old-time refrigerator. In the summer it was used to store milk, butter, eggs, and other perishables. The milk was kept in large crocks covered with wooden lids. In the winter, these were moved to the upstairs porch.

The floor of the cellar was hard dirt, almost like stone. A few burlap sacks were thrown here and there and in them or on them were stored potatoes, apples, and maybe turnips. On one side a few shelves held home-canned fruits and vegetables and jars of pickled vegetables, jellies, and preserves.

Dad had to toss in bed a couple of hours before he'd resort to the standard sleep-maker of those days — a glass of warm milk. It meant a trip to the cellar. He'd tiptoe out of the bedroom, light a hall candle, or kerosene lamp, and nobody would hear him until those squeaky cellar doors were pulled open.

Then Mom would pop up. Fearing a prowler, she would lean over to wake Dad and seeing he wasn't in bed, realized it was probably him. She'd put on a robe and by the time he closed those squeaky doors and arrived in the kitchen, she would have a fire in the stove.

"It's better if I warm it, and put some honey in."

"You havin' trouble sleepin', too?"

"Nobody can sleep with those cellar door hatches groanin' the way they do."

"Hm-m-m."

A SIMPLE STRETCH BEFORE RETIRING THAT HASTENS SLEEP

Tension is probably the most common cause of poor rest. If we can relieve tension in a natural way, then we should have a natural rest. Here is a stretching movement that helps relieve tension. It is helpful, though, only to the extent of the effort you exert.

It is simply performed:

1. Reach as high as possible.
2. Hold this position while standing on tiptoes with fingers outstretched as if reaching for the ceiling. Now count to thirty.
3. Slowly tighten the muscles of the arms, neck, chest, abdomen, hips, and legs as if holding onto an invisible heavy object.
4. Retain this tightened position bringing yourself downward to a squatting position.
5. Now press down on the floor with the hands for a count of thirty.
6. Let go.
7. Repeat this entire exercise three times.
8. Afterwards, shake the arms and legs. Then retire, and enjoy a good night's sleep.

Polly R., a secretary of 38 years of age, worked in a large office and was under heavy pressure caused by her busy routine.

Polly ate right, exercised, led a wholesome life in general, but had greatest difficulty trying to get her night's sleep.

She had used various preparations advertised for promoting sleep with little or no benefit. She had tried counting sheep and various other suggestions given to her by friends, but to no avail.

Upon examination and consultation, I could find nothing other than this clue: it was very difficult for her to leave her work at the office.

I treated her to give her more relaxation and instructed her in how to do this special stretching and tightening movement. Within three days after practicing this before retiring, Polly was able to go to sleep within a very short time. She felt more relaxed at work and found this to be the best old-fashioned remedy yet. I have used this movement and stretching procedure with any number of people, both young and old, with equally good results.

THINGS YOU CAN DO DURING THE DAY TO MAKE YOU SLEEP BETTER AT NIGHT

A cold shower to wake you up in the morning. A warm bath to relax you in the evening. This seems to be the standard accepted advice handed down through the generations.

There is certainly validity in the waking up effect of cold water. It is not due only to the shocking aspect, but physiologically speaking, when cold water chills the skin, it drives the blood away from those areas. Then a secondary reaction takes place: the superficial blood vessels expand, the blood returns to the surface, and circulation is stimulated.

As to the tepid or warm bath for the inducement of relaxation, since it is at skin temperature, the psysiological effects are confined to the mild hydro-therapy involved — contact with a massaging effect of the water. But this can be quite soothing and so I can perpetuate this advice in all good conscience.

On the other hand, there are those who remember how a cold compress used to be applied around the neck to induce sleep. A cloth was dipped in cold water, wrapped around the neck, and covered with a dry piece of wool or flannel. Its relaxing effect came, not when it was cold, but when it warmed up later, due to the containing of body heat by the covered compress.

Common sense has not changed much over the years, and it is still sensible to stay away from drinking stimulants like coffee or tea before bedtime. It is still sensible to eat lightly later in the day, having a big breakfast rather than a heavy dinner. It is still sensible to enjoy some mild physical activity before retiring, like an outdoor stroll. Yes, if you are thinking about sexual activity, that has been helping people to fall asleep for millennia.

One thing you can do during the day is not worry about whether you are going to be able to sleep that night. Some people enjoy keeping score. "I had only four hours of sleep last night, and three hours the night before. I sure have a lot of catching up to do tonight."

When these people get to bed, they are so concerned about whether they are going to fall asleep, they keep themselves up worrying about it.

THE ANATOMY OF SLEEP

An active mind is the opposite of a sleeping mind. However, do not interpret this to mean the sleeping mind is totally inactive. Far from that.

A generation or two ago, about all we knew on the subject of sleep was that a person was not conscious while asleep, that the movements were apparently an irrational series of grunts, groans, slurred words, tosses, turns, and an occasional yell.

Today we have more evidence of the nature of sleep. A biomedical device called the electroencephalograph (EEG) records a person's brain waves. A shift in these brain wave patterns is apparent when a person moves from the awake to sleep state. Generally speaking, this shift is from roughly twenty pulsations per second to five pulsations per second.

It has also been found that, while dreaming, a person's brain wave pulsations quicken to ten pulsations per second and that a rapid eye movement takes place (REM).

EEG reports of a quickening to ten pulsations per second coincide with observations of REM. This dreaming period comes in cycles, increasingly frequent as the night wears on.

Individuals deprived of the dreaming portions of the sleep cycle, by being awakened at their advent as shown in the EEG, will suffer mentally much more quickly than when deprived of the slower pulsation, non-dreaming parts of the sleep cycle. Apparently the dreaming aspect of sleep is an important function of the whole process.

Perhaps the most significant aspect of this research is not so much the identification of the brain wave rates at which sleep takes place, but the kinds of mental procedures that induce a lowering of brain wave frequency.

This lowering is caused by any kind of relaxation including various disciplines such as yoga, self-hypnotism, and meditation.

The act of merely closing your eyes begins this brain wave change. Taking a deep breath helps, both normal going-to-sleep preliminaries.

Visualizing a peaceful scene contributes to this lowering of the brain wave frequency. The time-worn practice of counting sheep thus wins some points as having validity.

Many of the commercial mind courses that assist people in being in more control of their lives use this principle in teaching sleep control techniques.

One example is Silva Mind Control, which uses a simple visualizing technique applied once a person has closed the eyes and relaxed the body. The person then imagines a blackboard and chalk. He mentally draws a circle, inside it a square, and inside the square the number 99. He then erases the number being careful not to erase the square or circle, successively writing in 98, 97, 96, etc. Most people fall asleep after writing just a few descending numbers.

If you prefer to count sheep, go ahead. It comes well recommended.

THE RIGHT WAY TO TIRE YOUR BODY FOR BETTER SLEEP

I mentioned earlier that one thing you can do during the day to aid your sleep is take a stroll in late afternoon or early evening. Any activity triggers the need for rest, but a mild activity is better than a violent activity. The violent activity works also, but it takes longer for the body to simmer down and accept sleep.

The American housewife is not doing the kind of hard muscle work that Grandma used to experience getting the chores done. And the average American male, especially urban male, is not getting the kind of tiring physical exercise that Grandpa found in a day's work.

Today's labor saving devices are costing some of us lost sleep. We do not tire ourselves. The dishwasher saves washing dishes and drying them. The electric can opener saves elbow grease. The sink disposal deprives us of that stroll out to the garbage can and back, — not to speak of the car, the office elevator, and electronic robots that do office and factory work for us.

I'm not saying you should sell the washer and revert to the scrub board, nor am I saying you should sell the car and walk to work. But I am saying you need to move the body around more and if you don't, you have no argument with the old sandman when he does not come around the moment you hit the hay.

Over a thousand years ago there lived a people who had the same problem, perhaps even worse. The Taoist monks of China meditated continuously. These wise men realized that their bodies needed the benefits of natural movement. So they developed Tai Chi, a series of movements based on the slow, natural movements of animals. A few minutes of Tai Chi would give every muscle in their body a motion treat. People are still doing Tai Chi today in China to relax, acquire a more youthful appearance, stimulate vitality, and sleep better at night. It is now becoming popular in other countries including those of the West.

You do not have to know Tai Chi in order to tire your body in a natural way to invite sleep.

You can invent your own movements. Take dancing. That is the kind of free, natural rhythmical movement that your body loves. No one to dance with? Then dance by yourself. Move around with or without music and "do your own thing." Feel the exhilaration of it as you flow with natural grace.

Or, if you are not a dancer by nature, move in some other ways. Try to avoid specialized movements contained by some rigid requirements. Bicycling, for example, may be good, but it gives more movement to below the hips; less to above the hips. Nature does not play favorites.

Rowing or paddling would be better. Here the whole body comes into play. And speaking of play, croquet, horseshoes, badminton, and other lawn games involve you in a number of different movements that are therapeutic for your body cells.

Avoid violent exercise, especially before retiring. Calisthenics are setting-up exercises, not settling-down exercises.

A few pressures I describe in this book fall into a category of exercises that are really not exercises as we used to understand the word. There is no motion in standing with your hands on your rib cage and exerting pressure. When you pit muscle against muscle, you are doing an isometric exercise.

Isometric exercises are a good way to tire the body to induce sleep. No running, no breathing hard, no sweating, no fuss, no exertion. You can devise your own isometric exercises, after I give you an example or two.

Put your palms together in hand clasp fashion in front of your chest. Now press one palm against the other. Keep up the pressure for a minute or two.

Stand alongside a wall, one shoulder touching it. Let the wrist and hand push on the wall, harder and harder. Now release the pressure and step away from the wall to relax. In the old days they would enjoy a laugh as the arm rose involuntarily a foot or two once pressure was released. Try it.

Two persons can do their isometric exercises together. Sit in opposite chairs, knees touching. Hold both palms out, touching. Now push. There is no desire to push the other person over, just to apply stationary pressure. Again, they used to make a game out of this by using one arm and a table. Each person would place his elbow on the table, arm vertical, hands clasped, and try to pressure the other to lower his hand.

These isometric exercises can be devised to give muscles practically anywhere in your body a chance to benefit. However, they are not meant to be a substitute for motion.

If you do isometric "exercises," take a nice walk, too.

IF YOU MUST TAKE A SLEEP REMEDY, THIS IS A HARMLESS ONE THAT WORKS

According to a panel of experts which conducted a three-year review of over twenty ingredients in nonprescription stimulants, sedatives, and sleep inducers, only one of these ingredients — caffeine — was found to be safe and effective. I'd rather not dwell on that ingredient, but prefer to note some of the other ingredients they looked into.

Take bromides. These are very toxic substances. Also scopolamine compounds. Both were found to be ineffective at currently marketed doses and not safe at doses that would be effective. In other words, if a person took more than the directions set forth, which is a common procedure when you want some medicine to work, that person could suffer serious damage.

My conclusion: Old-fashioned sleep remedies work best — and are safest.

Most sleeping pills on the market are unwise to use. I think I have already made myself clear about the damages of these chemicals.

However, there are some natural remedies for sleeplessness that are not harmful.

First, all of the herb teas that help calm the nerves, like valerian, as described in the previous chapter, also induce sleep, except of course regular tea which acts in reverse as a stimulant.

They had an herb lined up for every problem in the old days. Old herb books spell out remedies for catarrh, menstrual pain, ingrown toenails, even "running fits in dogs."

Health food stores still carry herbs that fill specific needs, including sleeplessness, which are not available at regular food stores. Many old remedies have survived through a brand of medicine known as homeopathy, founded in the eighteenth century. The name is derived from the Greek "homios" meaning "similar" and "pathos" meaning disorder. You might say it uses likes to treat likes. This is done by giving a small dose of something that causes the same symptoms as the complaint; a small dose is said to trigger the body's defenses more intensely.

What I personally like about the homeopathic philosophy is its use of natural substances. These do not create the dangerous side effects of many regular drugs which often do more harm than the original problem.

A homeopathic remedy for sleeplessness is one of the so-called cell salts, — mineral substances in the body that are essential nutrients. This one is phosphate of potash. It is a material found in just about all the body tissues and body fluids, but notably in the brain cells and nerve cells. Any company that sells homeopathic remedies stocks this one — obtainable without prescription.

Nervousness and sleeplessness are a possible indication that you have drained your body's nervous system of this salt through some emotional strain. Replenish it and sleep comes.

The natural foods that folks ate in the old days to calm the nerves and permit healthful sleep contained phosphorus among other nutrients, particularly milk, eggs, cheese (unprocessed), and meats (not of the sausage or cold cut variety). Phosphorus, calcium, and vitamin D are needed in balanced amounts in order to be properly utilized by the body.

We now get back to why Gramps made that trip to the root cellar to get milk. It's a balanced nerve tonic.

BODY POSITIONS AND THEIR EFFECT ON HEALTHFUL SLEEP

In Chapter 7, I discussed how in several cases, backaches were relieved by changing a person's sleeping position.

If you are sleeping in a position that is not conducive to total health, there is a good chance your subconscious mind might interfere with that sleep in order to get you to change your position. Once awake, your conscious mind takes over and you direct your body back to one of the familiar positions regardless of its propriety.

Ralph Martin, Doctor of Chiropractic, writes in *Healthways Magazine*,* that a large percentage of people with low-back disorders, as well as whiplash, bursitis, and neuritis of the shoulder, who fail to respond to treatment as well as might be expected have been found to lie in sleeping positions which tend to perpetuate their problems and pains.

I agree with Dr. Martin when he recommends that a serious study be made of how sleeping positions affect general health. We spend some one-third of every day in bed, if not in sleep, and if that time contributes in any way to musculo-skeletal strain or to blocked circulation or to nerve pressure, there are bound to be minus effects on health level.

Also, the matter of breathing is important. The first thing a mother is wary of for her newborn child is the freedom to breathe while in a crib position. In later months or years we may not suffocate, as we would awake and change our position, but we might not necessarily awake if that position was merely detracting from the optimum by placing a mild restriction on the diaphragm. Still, that distraction could cause health problems.

In Chapter 7, I told you how an on-the-stomach sleeping position can cause lower-back problems. In this position these muscles relax in such a way as to permit the spine to slip slightly forward.

---

*May, 1975.

On awakening you can feel it in your lower back. Correct this by sleeping on the side, knees drawn up.

This belly sleeping position is also troublesome to the neck and can produce a "kink" (with subluxation or partial dislocation); or, by partially blocking veins in the neck, can interfere with circulation to the head. It can also lead to bursitis because of the tendency in this position to raise the arm and use it for a pillow.

Two natural sleeping positions are: on the back, and on the side, knees drawn up.

How do you control your sleeping position? Remember, that if you are restless, awaking frequently, it may be because your subconscious wants you to assume a different healthier sleeping position.

On the other hand, if you are sleeping well, but awaking with a back, leg, or shoulder problem, instruct your subconscious to work for you. Here is how:

Relax after you climb into bed. Then talk to your subconscious mind. Give it a name if you find that is easy to do. One patient of mine calls his George. Say, "George, if I turn on my stomach while asleep, wake me up and let me remember the reason I am awaking."

Try it. It works. George is always awake and is listening.

HOW AN OLD-FASHIONED KITCHEN UTENSIL AIDS SLEEP

Did you ever hear of a rolling pin? Some people still have them to roll dough, but how many people today bake their own bread or pies? Nobody did it for you in the old days, unless you went to a county fair or church bake sale, so you needed a wooden rolling pin to flatten the dough.

Now you can put that wooden rolling pin to another useful purpose to help you sleep. It is not as far-fetched as it sounds. We talked about the usefulness of massage to help you relax. Massage of the feet is helpful to relax the entire body preparatory to sleep.

This should be performed in the evenings for best results. You don't need a rolling pin. You can rub the soles of the feet over the edge of a kitchen chair like Uncle Zeke used to do. You can leave your socks or stockings on, or take them off.

When Mr. J. R., machinist, came to me, his main complaint was that he could not sleep more than four hours a night, that he was almost exhausted from lack of rest, and that his feet especially felt tired.

He was instructed to use a wooden (not glass) rolling pin in his home by placing it on the floor, rolling his feet across this rolling pin, applying as much pressure as he could tolerate for three minutes on each foot. By practicing this therapy each night, within one week most of his tiredness was eliminated, and he was sleeping eight hours every night.

I have found foot massage so beneficial to my patients and rolling pins or chair rungs at best an improvisation, that I have invented and patented a foot massager. Although it is not yet manufactured and marketed, the prototype has been used safely by people of all ages, by themselves. It is not a vibrator or hydromassager like other products on the market. It pulsates, rotates, and kneads. This triple action on the sole of the foot aids relaxation and sleep as well as foot circulation and strength.

For some people, feet are at the bottom of the sleep problem and a good foot massage can mean a good night's sleep.

A SURPRISE BEVERAGE THAT INDUCES SLEEP

There is an animal on most farms that used to be used more commonly than it is today as a source of milk—the goat.

Goat's milk was frequently used to calm the stomach, such as cases of nervous indigestion, butterflies in the stomach, etc. Milk is a good food to begin with, but goat milk is an even better food and more easily digestible.

I have used goat milk for both young and elderly people who were allergic to cow's milk without any adverse reaction to the goat milk. The only complaint I have found is that some patients seem to think there is a stigma against using goat milk. For them, it affects the taste. To overcome this, I recommend the following:

2 tablespoons Carob Powder (*not* cocoa or chocolate)
1 tablespoon honey
1 pint goat milk

When mixed together in a blender, the above ingredients have a pleasantly rich, malt-like flavor.

As an example of the digestibility and soothing effect of goat milk, I cite the case of our infant son. It had been almost impossible to find a formula which would agree with him. He would seem to accumulate gas on several formulas.

At six weeks of age after drinking 1/3 to 1/2 bottle of formula, he would develop so much gas that he would practically jump out of his mother's arms. After changing to fresh goat milk (straight), he would drink the entire baby's bottle of goat milk and peacefully drop off to sleep.

It was unbelievable how quickly he adapted to the goat milk. And it was a great sleep aid to his parents, too.

I have taken several of my patients off sleeping pills and put them on goat milk instead. It seems to have some substance which acts as a sedative or perhaps it is richer in the calcium, phosphorus and vitamin D nerves require than even cow's milk is.

I remember one lady, in particular, who had a severe insomnia problem. When Mrs. E., 45, first came to me, she complained of not being able to sleep more than two or three hours out of any twenty-four hour period. She had suffered with this condition for several weeks and had been taking large amounts of codeine to no avail. She was treated and told to drink six ounces of goat's milk with each meal and at bedtime.

Within one week she was sleeping regularly eight peaceful hours per night.

10

COMMON AILMENTS YOU CAN GET RID OF UNCOMMONLY FAST NATURE'S WAY

In this chapter we are going to talk about common ailments, there being no more common ailment than the common cold, but we will be including such extensions of the common cold to the respiratory system as tonsilitis and sinus, and we will also look into what steps the country people used to take to combat asthma, influenza, and a few other ailments that were probably just as common then as they are today.

Winter was and is the time when colds strike, and during the fall months, the country folk still scurry around before the hard freeze digging rutabagas, chicory, parsnip, burdock, and other roots and storing them either in the root cellar or in some other accessible-in-the-snow spot where they would be covered with maple leaves or wood chips.

They squirrel away butternuts, hickory, and hazelnuts. They create an indoor greenhouse with an old apple crate or two, and plant watercress, dill, parsley, and onion grass. They hang the last cabbages from rafters and maybe mark with colored ribbons on sticks where other vegetables like lettuce and broccoli may later be found still growing beneath the snow.

There would be store food available all winter long. No fear of that. But here was nature's store of food and that was not only sustenance but protection from winter's challenge.

NATURE'S GROWING THINGS THAT HELP RELIEVE RESPIRATORY PROBLEMS

If these country folk knew their roots, herbs, and other natural, growing remedies, they would also mark where the wild asparagus grew, and they would gather some aconite bulbs if they could find them and surely some belladonna.

Today these remedies are available in some health food stores or from homeopathic supply firms. Aconite is helpful when the common cold is in its first stage. Perhaps the face is hot, but the rest of your body is cold, or perhaps you have a tickling in your throat and the beginnings of a cough.

Also at this stage, the rose hip is most effective. You may have picked these in late summer when they were at their ripest and dried them for just this occasion. Now their tea infuses your system with concentrated vitamin C, the vitamin that Linus Pauling confirmed is helpful in fighting off cold germs. Other research has confirmed that the blood's constables — the white blood corpuscles — do their policing more efficiently in an environment which is rich in ascorbic acid (vitamin C).

Gelsemium is recommended by many at the onset of flu when you are dulled by fever and chills.

Where there is frequent sneezing and discharge of mucus, arsenicum is often used or pulsatilla or allium cepa.

Although I was not there when it happened, the story is told of the famous opera singer who woke up on the morning of her big performance with a sore throat and a rasping voice.

Frantic, she called her manager, but that only made matters worse, as he practically lost his voice in his frustration and frenzy. A few hours before the scheduled performance she remembered something her mother had used — raw onion. Her manager brought her some. She took a large one, chopped it up into pieces and then ate them, chewing carefully, and swallowing until the whole onion was gone. That night she hit high C with her usual ease, and the opera was a success, and nobody suspected the problem — except maybe the first row.

I do remember a cough remedy they used to use made of onion. The grated onion was covered with honey and baked until the juice oozed from it. Then it was taken in tablespoon doses to relieve not only a cough but also asthma.

Garlic is in more common use today in this respect. Rich in organic iodine, it is used as a natural septic for the body. It cleanses the digestive tract of germs and also the blood. The juice of garlic is used for sore throats, hoarseness, and asthma.

A doctor has to be courageous to recommend onions or garlic to anybody for anything. I prefer a gentler course.

THE OLD-FASHIONED WAY TO CHECK COLD SYMPTOMS THAT IS MOST EFFECTIVE

Even though there is no cure for colds or flu, from which everyone has suffered then and now, the old timers used a few simple aids that effectively helped to check the symptoms, or at least make them more bearable.

At the onset when you feel like you are catching cold:

1. Take hot sweat baths. Recline in the bathtub. Cover your body with water as warm as can be tolerated. As you become accustomed to this temperature, gradually add warmer water until you notice perspiration forming on your forehead.
2. Upon leaving the bathtub, drink a hot lemonade, flavored with honey. (Lemons are a good source of vitamin C). Then rest in bed covered with blankets to promote further perspiration.
3. Irrigate the sinus with saline solution as described later in this chapter.
4. For sore throat, gargle with one part apple cider vinegar mixed with two parts warm water. Do this hourly or as needed.
5. For coughs, mix one part lemon juice to one part honey. Take one tablespoon every hour, or as needed.
6. Body elimination is important. If you fail to have your regularly normal bowel movement, take an enema using plain, body temperature water. If fever persists, take this enema hourly.

7. Avoid solid foods including eggs (egg whites especially), cow's milk, and any other mucus forming foods. (Some authorities now feel that citrus fruits in large quantities could be mucus forming). Concord grape juice is recommemded for restoring strength and as cold symptoms wane. Drink as much as desired.

Said one man in his fifties who had suffered countless colds in his life, "Doctor, that system of yours works. I was rid of those cold symptoms in forty-eight hours. I believe that's one cold I never really had."

GRANDMOTHER'S COLD PREVENTION REMINDERS

Hardly a winter starts without some authority being quoted in the newspapers, on television, or through some other media on how many people will catch colds in the months ahead and how many work hours will be lost. Or, perhaps there is a new influenza virus on the march and trouble is expected.

These scare tactics are dangerous in that they can bring on what they are alerting you to. Fear and anxiety about anything lowers the body resistance.

When grandmother made a few cautionary observations she did not mean to be a worry wart and there was no threat of disease in her tone, but rather a promise of continued good health.

The wise observations she shared are still valuable today. Certainly if we took the time to observe some of her time-tested advice many of these hours of sniffly discomfort would be avoided.

What did grandmother advise? Well, let's let her speak through me now:

- Dress warmly in cold weather. That means even if you are just going to the barn for a minute, or next door.
- Remove heavy outer clothing as soon as you are back indoors. Even if you expect to go right out again, it is all the more reason to remove these outer garments so you don't begin to perspire.
- Change wet clothes right away. Drying them out on you saps your body heat and strength. Replace damp clothing or socks with dry clothing promptly.
- Don't over-exert yourself. Overworking and over-playing add an energy drain on your body at a time of the year

when extreme temperature changes are putting an added load on the body's normal functions.

- Respect body signals. If you feel tired, let go. Don't be a hero. Give in to your body's protestations. It knows what is good for you. Spend the rest of the day relaxing with a good book.

It is hard for a doctor to tell his patients any of these things without sounding like his mother or his grandmother. The reason it is familiar is because it is common sense passed on from family to family and generation to generation.

"Feed a cold, starve a fever" is an old adage. I do not know when or where it got started, but I think letting up on food today is a help to combating a cold as well as a fever. It is only a mild cold that is free of fever, so what they may be saying is the same as what I am saying — the worse the situation, the less you eat the better off you'll be.

Every doctor gets into trouble telling his patients to eat less. That's why most doctors don't like to wrestle with obesity cases. I guess I am just as timid as the rest.

However, when the parent brings a child in with cold symptoms, the way is clear. Tell the parent and let the parent wrestle with the child.

I have treated a great number of children who have had colds and tonsilitis. My suggestion has always been to the parent to take the child off milk, heavy starches, and sweets, substituting large amounts of fruit juice, with Concord grape juice as first choice, and, secondly, apple juice or apple cider. I have re-examined children two to three days after making this dietary change, and found their tonsils reduced to normal size and of normal color, and cold symptoms relieved.

A SIMPLE HOME REMEDY FOR SINUS CONGESTION

The stuffed-up nose, for most people a passing symptom of the common cold, can for some people be a chronic condition that is at once troublesome and enervating.

When the sinus area becomes irritated, mucus forms that can fill the nasal cavity and seriously impede breathing.

A number of remedies for sinus have been used in the past with varying success — like horseradish, which was grated and taken in small fractions of a teaspoon, with lemon juice, several times a day. Prepared horseradish today may not be as effective as freshly made horseradish.

Also, onions taken the same way the opera singer used them helps to loosen mucus and to drain sinus cavities.

But the old-fashioned tried-and-true remedy with which I have had the best results is a normal saline solution. That's right: nature's own salt water.

If you are not near the ocean, or even if you are but prefer kitchen convenience, common table salt in water is just as effective, but water should be distilled.

To prepare, thoroughly dissolve one rounded teaspoon of table salt in one pint of tepid water. Using distilled water is important, as many water sources contain chlorine, etc., which are very irritating to tender sinuses. After cupping this solution into the palm of the hand, hold it to the nose and breathe in. Tip the head backward so that the solution can be drawn into the throat; then spit out the solution. A very inexpensive aspirator (nasal syringe) will do a better job. Most pharmacies or similar retail stores sell these.

Repeat this procedure morning and evening, taking care not to draw in the solution too harshly.

Some people have accepted their difficulty in breathing as a way of life. But then other disorders can arise as a result of it.

Mrs. A. L., age 40, had suffered from migraine headaches for six years. Sedation had had no effect whatsoever. Upon examining the patient, I found her condition was basically sinusitis.

She was given the recommendation to eliminate all highly seasoned, spicy foods as well as mucus forming foods, such as cow's milk and eggs. She was instructed to sniff a normal saline solution twice daily for two minutes. Within one week her headaches were completely alleviated, and she was breathing "better than I can remember."

A MASSAGE THAT AIDS SINUS AND HEADACHE

Sinus and headache are frequent companions. They can make the sunniest of days appear to be dull and the most joyful days a drag.

Either can be persistent or recurrent. Either by itself can be a nuisance. Together they make a disabling team.

When one has a headache, painful sinus, or eye discomfort, a great amount of relief may frequently be obtained by using the massage.

By massaging the temples and across the forehead above the eyes you will help to relax the facial nerve, relieving the tightly drawn areas of the face.

THESE HAND MASSAGES CAN RELIEVE A MIGRAINE HEADACHE

Another effective massage is based on nerve endings that occur in the feet and in the hands. Pressure on the nerve endings in the palm can relieve persistent headache.

Merely take the thumb of one hand and press the palm of the other. Press as firmly as you can. If there is pain in the palm from pressing this is all the more reason that this pressure needs to be applied *(Figure 10-1)*.

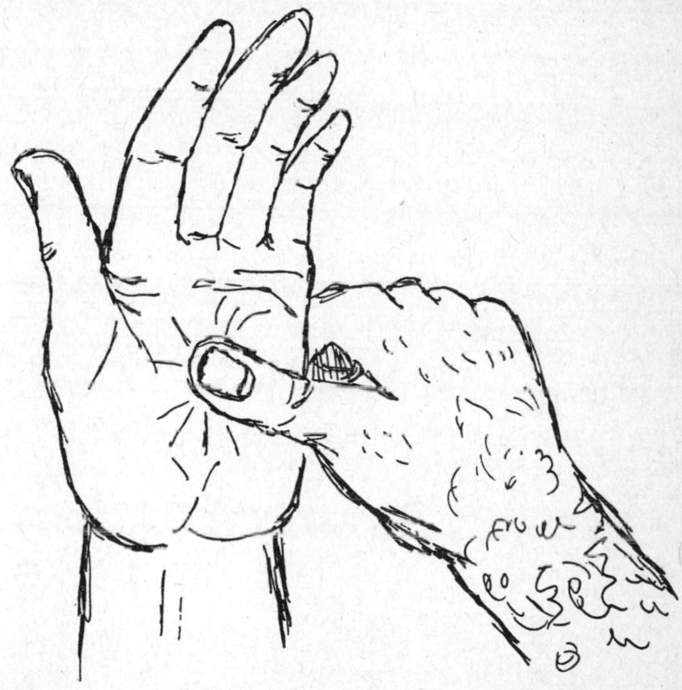

Figure 10-1

Hand Massages

Another spot on the hand where nerve endings affect headache is the second joint of the thumb. Use oil or hand lotion on the thumb, to lessen friction. Then, using the thumb and index finger of the other hand, rub this joint vigorously.

Repeat the process switching thumbs. If the headache is very severe, ten minutes of hard, vigorous massage on each thumb (with oil) may be required.

Mrs. G. had suffered with migraine headaches for the past thirteen years. She had received slight relief from various medications. They reduced the severity but not the headaches in entirety. The treatments I gave her in the office would sometimes completely relieve the headache for as much as two or three days, but the headaches would come back later.

I instructed her in this hand massage therapy, using it when she felt even the slightest headache coming on.

Soon she could go a week or two weeks and then up to three or four months without a headache. This remedy has been used by many of my patients successfully. If the migraine sufferer will use this, he should get a good degree, if not complete relief, in the control of his headaches.

I love to see the expression on the faces of my disbelieving patients as the thumb or palm is massaged and the headache gradually recedes — pleasure mixed with wonder, as though some kind of miracle has taken place.

A word about another way to relieve headache pain. In those parts of the country and at those times of the year when strawberries are available, you have a natural pain-killer. Strawberries are one of the few foods that contain organic salicylates similar to the active ingredients of aspirin. The frozen variety, no sugar added, if available, would also be effective.

A WAY TO HELP CHEST TENSION AND ASTHMA

There is a groundswell of national interest today in non-drug, non-surgery methods of natural healing. It is partially due to the high cost of medical disciplines, partially due to their abuse or misuse resulting in malpractice suits, in turn resulting in high insurance premiums for doctors and still higher costs to the patient.

It is also partially due to the realization that one drug leads to another and seldom does the path lead out of the woods.

On the other hand, natural healing methods hardly ever have side effects that in turn require treatment. Natural healing methods may not be as swift or dramatic, and they may not even work at all, if the right materials or methods are not hit upon.

But still they are *safe* and *inexpensive.* These are the two factors that contribute to the surge of interest, or, if you will, return of interest in the old-fashioned, natural ways.

I remember hearing a New England farmer tell about how his grandmother helped him stop wheezing. He now thinks this is probably what they call asthma today.

At any rate, she used cranberries. Yup, you heard me right — those tasty red berries that most of us forget about all year till that holiday turkey is served again.

She would mash some cranberries through a strainer and add some warm water. A cup of this would cause an almost immediate opening of the bronchial tubes.

Now it has been found that cranberries contain an ingredient that acts as a bronchial antispasmodic. It dilates the bronchial tubes in the same way that adrenalin or other drug a doctor may inject into the bloodstream works, without the pollution of the system and the weakening of natural body resistance that this causes.

Cranberries are not necessarily a cure for asthma, but neither is the adrenalin or other drug used for relief. Cranberries can be a more healthful, natural relief.

No real cure for asthma was ever handed down from previous generations. Today we realize that asthma is an emotionally caused condition. More about ways to relieve psychosomatic disorders in the final chapter of this book. Asthma's particular emotional cause appears to have something to do with an overly possessive kind of parental love. You might call it "smother love."

The fact is, when children who have asthma are sent away to a clinic for treating, the best treatment they receive is getting away from smother love. They are practically cured when they get on the train or plane. Then when there is a visit again with parents — relapse.

Here is a way used years ago to relax the diaphragm for healthful, deep breathing. It is helpful in cases of asthma as well as chest congestion and chest colds. When you fill the lungs to their maximum you help detoxify the body. This is a hand pressure method, performed quite simply.

1. While standing, place both hands with fingers pointing forward upon the lower ribs.
2. Press inward as far as the ribs will allow with both hands at the same time, exhaling with the mouth open.
3. Suddenly release both hands at the same time.
4. Inhale deeply.
5. Breathe in and out to a steady count so that in breaths take the same time as out breaths.

Three to six times of pressure and release are usually sufficient before you do your deep breathing for a few minutes.

One youngster who had suffered from asthma for six years was instructed in this hand-rib pressure followed by deep, even breathing three times daily and told to use it at school whenever he felt an asthmatic attack coming on. Within six weeks this youngster made a great recovery. He was not completely free of asthma, but he now could control the problem. The family later moved away, and I could not get a further follow-up on this case.

In years gone by when a person in the family suffered from occasional asthmatic attacks, he or she was asked by the older folk to do certain breathing exercises. These were basically to restore conscious control.

Today we have biofeedback equipment that helps with such extension of the conscious mind over subconscious-controlled functions. At Children's Memorial Hospital in Chicago, asthmatic children have been "taught" to prevent and shorten asthmatic attacks. In the experimental program, the children breathed into an apparatus which measured the volume of exhaled air. They relaxed and tried to increase the volume and were rewarded when they did.

The children so trained had fewer attacks, some reduced by ninety percent, and required less medication. It became automatic for the muscles to relax whenever the bronchial tubes began to have spasms, thus permitting the tubes to dilate, or open wider.

In chiropractic we ask, "What causes these bronchial tube contractions?" The answer is that it is a muscular movement triggered by an abnormal nerve impulse. So we address ourselves to the abnormality or irritation of these nerves that supply nerve energy to the small bronchi.

In both cases the same cause is treated. In the biofeedback equipment, conscious control is exerted to correct the abnormal nerve impulses. In chiropractic, normality is restored to these nerve impulses.

A LONG FORGOTTEN SUBSTANCE THAT RELIEVES CHEST TENSION

Did you ever hear of snuff? You can still get it in tobacco stores and some large pharmacies. It used to be as common as a loaf of bread.

The memory of snuff that most of us have is that of a bewigged English nobleman reaching into his vest pocket, removing a jeweled snuff-box, placing a little of this dust-like material on his fingers, placing them to his nose, breathing in quickly, pausing, and then producing a bellowing sneeze that obviously gave him a great deal of pleasure.

Sneezes are good for the lungs since they exercise the rib cage, diaphragm, and help the respiratory system in general.

An irritant to the nasal passages — whether it be a cold breeze or a foreign substance — usually causes a sneeze or a series of sneezes. The increase in the volume of air in the lungs is a benefiting factor.

Relief from chest tension by means of a few healthy sneezes can be accomplished simply. Take a small pinch of snuff and inhale in the nose. Before breakfast is usually the best time. The sneezing will take place almost immediately, and you will be surprised how much better you will feel and how much of your chest tension will disappear, milord.

Yes, milady uses snuff, too, but only in the privacy of her boudoir.

Care should be taken not to overuse snuff. It might set up too much irritation in the nasal passage or possibly even a snuff addiction.

S. L., age 20, had a history of pleurisy. He would arise in the mornings with a tightness in his chest and difficulty in breathing. Although the pleurisy had run its course and the lung tissue had healed, he was left with these symptoms. To relieve this tension he was instructed to take a pinch of snuff into his nostrils on arising and sneeze vigorously. A week later upon arising he could breathe normally without the aid of the snuff. This provided a greater amount of relief for this young man than any previous therapy he had tried.

If you are concerned about shortness of breath and are starting to think in terms of maybe you have emphysema, here is a test you can do at home that could either send you to the phone to make an appointment with your doctor, or set your mind at ease.

Light a match and hold it three inches away from your mouth. Now, without taking a breath, blow it out.

If you succeed, you have plenty of residual air in your lungs, meaning that there are healthy air cells in your lung tissue working for you.

If, on the other hand, you have to draw in a breath to blow out the match you may want your doctor to check you. This means the resident air is not sufficient, or certainly below normal.

SOME TIPS FOR GETTING RID OF SUCH PROBLEMS AS RINGWORM, SCABIES, AND WARTS

Sometimes the bacteria, viruses, or other invaders of our bodies, instead of internal problems such as colds and flu, cause external or skin problems.

In Colonial days, they used the radish to get rid of warts. The radish was sliced and the warts rubbed several times a day with the white innards of the raddish.

Nobody has come to me with wart problems. I guess these days people learn to live with warts until they disappear on their own account. But I do see plenty of cases or ringworm.

Ringworm is not a worm, it's a fungus. It causes circular scaly patches on the skin and can be spread from one person to another. It is something like athlete's foot in that this, too, is a fungus and causes lesions. These lesions can be either dry and scaly or filled with fluid.

Any fungus, once it gets a hold on an area of your skin, can be a pretty stubborn invader. Common cold germs are attacked by the bloodstream where white blood corpuscles make short shrift of the invaders.

However, a fungus is a parasite that lives on your skin largely out of reach of the body's defenses. Treatment needs to be from the outside.

Jimmy H., age nine, was brought to my office with a ringworm on the top of his scalp. He had been afflicted with it for six weeks to two months. The condition was spreading quite rapidly, and he had lost a sizeable amount of hair in one spot. The previous therapies had not slowed down the spreading or promoted any healing. The previous doctor had told the mother of the boy that if her son's ringworm did not show signs of healing within one more week, he was going to use X-ray (radiation) treatment. This statement frightened the mother.

I instructed the mother to use a home treatment consisting of the application of a gauze saturated in a normal saline solution (one teaspoon salt dissolved in one pint of distilled water), followed the next day by applying another gauze pad saturated with a solution of one part vinegar mixed with four parts of distilled water. It was recommended that she should alternate these solutions daily. Within ten days the ringworm lesion was completely healed, and small hair was beginning to appear on his scalp.

That poor fungus. It had to contend with salt one day, acid the next. Salt, acid, salt, acid. It just figured there must be an easier scalp elsewhere.

I have used this same shock treatment on scabies, even though we are no longer talking about plant life, but a tiny eight-legged mite of the arachnid spider family. The insect burrows under the superficial layers of the skin and causes itching.

It appears as itchy red bumps, particularly between the fingers and near elbows, knees, abdomen, and genital areas. It is contagious and is often diagnosed incorrectly as another skin condition which it can often resemble.

Scabies come in twenty-year cycles. Prompt treatment is recommended — applications as for ringworm. And grandma laundered the clothes and bedding in boiling hot water to prevent spreading.

No, mites do not like a salt, acid, salt treatment either.

The balance in nature is beautiful to behold. For every scourge there is a remedy. Man has been through it all. All you have to do is find somebody who remembers.

11

DIGESTIVE AND ELIMINATION PROBLEMS THAT RESPOND TO THESE SAFE HOME REMEDIES

This would probably be voted as the most important chapter in the book were there to be a popularity contest. Stomach and intestinal problems are universal.

In the days of butter churns, corsets with stays, celluloid collars, and kerosene lamps, people had digestive and elimination problems, too. And just because these were also the days of bangs made of feathers to hide women's thinning hair and glass eyes for horses, it does not mean that they did not have effective home remedies for the upset stomach and the sluggish or obstreperous bowel.

They were not only effective, they were safe — compared to some of the things that we put in our stomach today in the name of stomach relief. Some of the antacids or pain-killers that we consume can cause far more trouble if taken frequently than the disorders we take them for.

The stomach is an incredible chemical laboratory, transforming food and food combinations, no matter how strange or complicated, into usable, absorbable material.

The key digestive substance is the enzyme.

THE KEY FACTOR IN GOOD DIGESTION

An enzyme is an internal juice formed by the cells of the digestive system. It is not actually used up in the digestive process, but rather acts as a catalyst, causing a chemical reaction to take plaçe without itself being changed or destroyed.

If it were not for enzymes, wine would not ferment, seeds would not sprout, and tobacco would not cure.

Enzymes make leaves change color in autumn, tomatoes turn from a unripe green to a tempting ripened red, and bananas assume their ready-to-eat golden color.

Different enzymes work in different foods. One might work on sugar and break it up into usable form; it is called sucrase. Another enzyme might work on phosphorous; it is called phosphatase.

The most important enzyme in the digestive process is pepsin. It works on protein that we eat, breaking it up into usable amino acids. Here are some other important enzymes:

- Rennin causes the coagulation of milk, releasing its phosphorous, calcium, potassium, and iron.
- Lipase splits fat
- Phyalin, contained in saliva, breaks down starch into usable maltose.

There are many enzymes stored in the liver, in the pancreas, and in the glands that nest in the mucous lining of the stomach. All help to extract vital nutrients from the food we eat for absorption by the bloodstream and utilization by cells throughout the body.

Foods that provide these enzymes are nature's digestion boosters.

TWO FRUITS FROM HAWAII THAT AID DIGESTION

Mrs. L. O., 70 plus years of age, had suffered with gastric disturbance for many years. She had taken various digestive preparations and nothing seemed to really help.

She was instructed to take one ounce of pineapple juice mixed with one ounce of papaya juice (or papaya concentrate) with each meal as a home treatment.

Thirty days later she returned to my office feeling and looking much better. She reported she had had very little, if any, gas after her meals since using this preparation.

This natural digestive aid has been used by many people with very gratifying results. The enzyme, papain, which is found in papaya, and the enzyme, bromelain, found in pineapple, are the digestive boosters.

Often the patient suffers from over-acidity. The body in its attempt to compensate for a lack of digestive enzymes in the diet secretes more acids. Then we have what we call over-acidity.

The doctor frequently prescribes an antacid for neutralizing the excess acid, which sometimes makes matters worse, as the body tries to compensate and puts out more acid.

By using bromelain (the pineapple enzyme) and papain (the papaya enzyme) we inhibit to a degree the excessive acids by supplying the proper enzyme for digestion. In effect, we correct the over-acidity.

Papaya has been around for a long time, even though many of us have been enjoying the taste of it recently for the first time. That is because it is a delicate fruit and difficult to ship over long distances.

Ancient explorers wrote about papaya frequently. Marco Polo said it cured his sailors of scurvy. Columbus reported on its great value when he returned to Spain. Ponce de Leon told how the natives he met used papaya and called it *vanti,* meaning, "keep well."

Papaya has such human characteristics as being of two sexes, there being male and female plants, and taking nine months for its embryo fruit to develop fully.

Natives hang tough meat in the papaya tree and it becomes more tender, or they wrap it in the leaves of the papaya tree. After festive banquets, they eat the papaya fruit to help digest the extra food. For generations, commercial meat tenderizers have used papain, extracted from papaya, as their active ingredient.

Papaya is found in almost every tropical area. With improved methods of air shipment, Hawaii papaya growers are now providing increased quantities of papaya to the principal cities.

I recommend papaya, or extract of papaya, available in most large food stores, for your improved digestion. It will not only help to relieve stomach distress, sluggishness, and heartburn, but when digestion improves, your whole body benefits.

Pineapple is another enzyme-rich fruit and in more general distribution. It contains bromelain which appears to act similarly to the pancreatic secretion, trypsin. There is a high chlorine content which helps to replace hydrochloric acid used in digestion.

Pineapple is imported to the American mainland largely from Hawaii and from Puerto Rico, although it grows in Florida. Each plant, with long, sword-like leaves, grows about three feet high and bears just one spiny fruit.

Extracts from pineapple and papaya — the juice or concentrate — make an excellent digestive team.

Perhaps this is one of the reasons why Hawaiians live longer than other Americans. In Hawaii, the average life span is 73.6 years or three years longer than the national average of 70.7 years, according to latest census figures.

FRUIT AND VEGETABLE JUICES THAT MAKE YOUR DIGESTIVE ORGANS REJOICE

According to *Natural Health World* magazine, if you weigh 160 pounds, you consist of

100 pounds of water
29 pounds of protein
25 pounds of fat
5 pounds of minerals
1 pound of carbohydrates

plus one quarter ounce of vitamins.

Now that would seem the vitamins are relatively unimportant; however, they keep the rest of us functioning.

But look at that water! We are like a Venice. Is there any wonder that liquids bearing gifts find their way quickly to where those gifts are needed?

Fruit and vegetable juices are indeed liquids bearing gifts.

Take the venerable apple. Eighty-five percent water, apples begin their benefits the minute we take that crisp bite and start chewing by stimulating the alkaline saliva flow to keep our mouth and breath clean and fresh.

I've already sung the praises of apples in earlier chapters. Not only are they an old-fashioned home remedy, but they will probably be a remedy of the future, too, as scientists discover more and more about the apple that confirms our forefathers' trust in it.

Several years ago, Michigan State University did a comprehensive study on the apple in a truly effective way. Biochemists can dissect the apple molecules and shrug their shoulders at what they identify. But the apple still does things for people and that is the approach the University took.

They studied five hundred students who ate two or three apples a day and compared them to a group that ate no apples. Here are the ways in which the apple eaters compared:

- Fewer colds and upper respiratory infections
- Fewer skin problems
- Fewer headaches and less nervousness
- Better ability to concentrate
- Less stomach and intestinal troubles

The latter benefit is our concern in this chapter. Apples have a regulating effect on the entire digestive system. Their work is so comprehensive that it is difficult to dissect the apple and say that this ingredient helps this and that ingredient helps that.

I would vote for the apple's pectin, a complex colloidal substance, a digestion aid, and its phosphorous, an enzyme, as its chief components that aid digestion. Pectin yields uronic acid which helps the body to get rid of toxins. But then its roughage or bulk aids elimination and there are other benefits in between.

When you juice the apple, you eliminate the cellulose bulk that aids bowel elimination, but you concentrate the other "goodies" and they are able to take a faster ride along your liquid communicators to the source of need.

Other juices work the same way. Here are a few that are especially helpful to the digestive and elimination system:

Carrot Juice — Has a soothing influence on ulcers, colitis, and other conditions involving an inflamed or sensitive stomach or intestinal lining. Reduces the putrifying factors in the colon. Good alkalizer.

Cabbage Juice — Contains an anti-peptic ulcer factor now tentatively identified as Vitamin U, found mostly in the loose outside leaves rather than in the head.

Endive Juice — Also called chicory and escarole, the green, curly leaves yield a juice that relieves acidosis, aids constipation, and stimulates the flow of bile.

Celery Juice — Leaves a source of calcium and sodium, stalks of potassium. Helps with hyperacidity, indigestion, and appetite. Also an aid in combating obesity.

Garlic Juice — A good intestional antiseptic which stimulates gastric juices and digestive activity. Do not take alone, mix with other juices like celery.

Spinach Juice — A blood enricher and gland regulator, is an efficient alkalizer and laxative. It is useful in relieving dyspepsia.

Rhubarb Juice — Stimulates the flow of bile. Aids constipation due to indigestion. Helps heal hemorrhoids and halt diarrhea. Not recommended where acidity exists and such other disorders as rheumatism, gout, arthritis, stones, and certain skin conditions.

Coconut Juice — Almost a complete food. The juice is bland and soothing in cases of stomach ulcers, gastritis, and colitis. High vitamin B content helps with digestive disorders.

Cranberry Juice — Natural acids assist digestion. Bowels are normalized, with both diarrhea and constipation corrected.

Grape Juice — Grape juice stimulates bile secretion, helps the body burn off excess fat, and is a mild laxative. It is a good blood cleanser and body builder in general, also an aid to nervousness because of its vitamin B.

Pear Juice —	Used for many years to aid digestion and relieve colitis. A mild laxative and tends to decrease urine acidity.
Lemon Juice —	A good cleanser to start the day with. Avoid using when inflammation of the stomach or intestines exists, but effective for acidosis, nausea, and biliousness.

These are the main vegetables and fruits other than the apple, papaya, and pineapple already mentioned. I did not list a vegetable like kale because it is less common than cabbage juice to which it is chemically similar. Nor did I list a vegetable like Jerusalem artichoke, a tuber which can yield nearly a pint of juice for each pound of vegetables, a juice which is beneficial to the digestive system. Jerusalem artichokes are one of nature's important health remedies, especially good for diabetes, but not that common to be placed in the above very brief listing.

A TREASURE FOR HEALTH AT THE BOTTOM OF THE SEA

Most Americans would stare at you in astonishment if you suggested they eat seaweed. Yet people on seacoasts all over the world find rich nutrition in this deep sea delicacy.

Ancient Hawaiians called seaweed *limu* and found scores of edible varieties. They could live on a diet of just poi, limu, and fish. Japanese have been collecting it and drying seaweed for easier use and making it a part of gourmet meals. I'll give you a recipe in a minute.

When we think how the rains have washed our topsoil into the sea for millions of years, we realize how the ocean beds are the most fertile growing areas on earth.

Seaweed sometimes grows over miles deep below the ocean surface. The leaves are known as dulse and used extensively in Scotland and Ireland as an additive to many dishes.

Trace minerals are named because only a trace goes a long way and usually only a trace can be found in the chemical composition of our growing foods. However, trace minerals are found in relative abundance in seaweed. Nutritionally speaking, it is like finding gold veins and ten-karat diamonds.

Dulse and kelp, dried seaweed, are available from health food stores. I recommend they be standard table items as they are better for you and your digestion than pepper and salt.

To say kelp is good for the digestion would be, in a way, inaccurate. Kelp is good for you. Where digestive juices are not being formed by the body in sufficient quantity to perform the digestive process thoroughly, some elements or trace minerals could be in short supply. If this is so, seaweed can furnish what is missing.

Seaweed is an excellent source of organic iodine, so important for metabolism. Not just the thyroid, but every gland in your body can benefit from seaweed.

If you would like to collect seaweed, be sure to check with a local fisherman as to which are the edible varieties. Once gathered, clean it, break it into small pieces, pour boiling water over it. After letting it drain for a minute, rinse in cold water, put in plastic bags and freeze. You then have a supply of nutritious seaweed which you can use from time to time in salad, with fish or as a relish.

To make a seaweed relish take sugar, salt, and Japanese vinegar, add chopped round onions and the seaweed.

Let your body relish it.

THE OLD-FASHIONED WAY TO STAY THIN AND WHY IT WORKS EVEN BETTER TODAY

Even though they were a more active people, our grandfolks still got fat. In those days, obesity was more a sign of middle age than it is today. Now overweight plays no age preferences. In those days, when you reached middle age, it meant you could afford farm hands to do the heavy chores, or else your own children were big enough to take these strenuous tasks off your hands.

As the heavier work was taken out of your hands, the heavier weight appeared on your girth.

What would the family doctor say in those days? "Agatha, you better cut down on the sweets and starches."

And so Agatha passed up her second portion of potatoes and stopped baking a pie in the middle of the week, just one on weekends.

Today sweets and starches are as much a part of twentieth

century progress as computers and satellites. To cut down on sweets and starches means to give up:

- Bottled or canned soda and other sweet drinks
- Beer and most mixed drinks
- Cake, cookies, pie, breads, rolls, pastries
- Spaghetti and pastas
- Candy
- Ice cream
- Potato chips and similar packaged snacks

What's left? You ask.

Unfortunately, not much — in terms of goodies that have become habitual with us.

Part of their good from our viewpoint is the speed with which we can go from thought to mouthful — not waiting for the oven to get hot or the batter to set — everything instantly available.

What is left — the things that are good for us — take a little more time. These I need not remind you again are the fruits, the vegetables, the cheeses, eggs, nuts, meats, fish, and poultry.

They take a little more time to prepare than a chocolate fudge sundae, but you add a lot more time to your life — years.

EATING HABITS THAT CONTRIBUTE TO NORMAL WEIGHT AND TROUBLE-FREE DIGESTION

Robert S., a young farmer, came to my office with the complaint that he thought he had stomach ulcers. I found he had been gulping down his noon and evening meals in five minutes flat and explained to him that he could not possibly have good digestion by eating in this manner.

"If you do not change your eating habits, you could have far more complications than ulcers," I warned.

After a couple of weeks both of seeing him in my office and of his eating more leisurely, he reported no more problems with his so-called ulcers. Poor eating habits are bad habits we all should never practice. I feel it is much better to miss a meal occasionally than to eat in this manner.

In the old days, a meal was an event.

Today we eat to get it over with. Breakfasts and lunches are particularly abused by eating on the run.

Gracious settings used to be the order of the day — folded napkins in rings, butter paddled into balls, fresh flowers, and a lit candle on the table.

Today we use paper napkins, put the butter out still wrapped in the paper it came in, and there's a permanent plastic flower arrangement on the table.

There used to be a moment of silence at the start of a meal in which thoughts turned away from the busyness and were calmed in a spirit of togetherness. Today we dig right in without losing a phrase in the conversation, even though it may be argumentative or about tense and difficult subjects.

We might not know the difference. But our stomach does. Digestive juices begin with the saliva, and if that gets short shrift because you need to swallow quickly so you can get your words out faster, then your digestion is off to a poor start and subsequent juices have to work harder.

Chewing slowly helps you to enjoy your food. You can eat less and weigh less when you enjoy each mouthful more. Chewing slowly breaks down the food into more easily saturated particles, so the bile and other juices can do a more efficient job with less of themselves required in the process.

Summing up, here are my principles for trouble-free, slenderizing, healthful eating. If they sound old-fashioned, you know why:

- Make meals a time of leisurely enjoyment
- Eat slowly, chewing well.
- Avoid fried, fatty foods, cooking and eating so as to minimize animal fat intake.
- Include meat, fish, cheese, or poultry in your menu at least one meal a day.
- Enjoy some fruits or vegetables in every meal.
- Eat some raw fruit or vegetable once every day.
- Minimize sweets and starches.
- Avoid prepared products that are likely to have the good cooked out, or chemical preservatives added.

ULCERS AND HEMORRHOIDS – THE PRICE OF MODERN DAY WORRYING AND FRUSTRATION

Ulcers are sores on the lining of the stomach or duodenum – the entrance to the upper intestines. They are apparently caused by the erosion of stomach acids. Since the stomach is protected by mucus and other oily substances, the question arises: what causes this protection to be insufficient for some people?

The answer came quite unexpectedly a few decades ago when a man was operated on for intestinal trouble and an aperture created which would take some time to heal. A "window" was placed in this aperture temporarily so that doctors could observe his progress.

One day, while a doctor was observing his stomach, the man got mad. Instantly his stomach lining became visibly irritated by stomach acids. From that time on we have had new insight into the role emotions play in our health. And we have been able to point the finger of balance in the case of ulcers to worry and anxiety specifically.

Hemorrhoids are swellings or dilations of the veins in the anal region. They manifest first as an itching which then becomes a painful mass of bleeding tissue.

It has been thought to be caused by sedentary occupations. But then heavy laborers get hemorrhoids, or piles as they are also known. It has been thought to be caused by constipation and the straining of muscles necessiated by this condition, but then diarrhea can also bring on piles. It has also been thought to be due to our diet of low residue (or low bulk) foods. This seems to have some merit and I'll discuss this in a moment.

The emotional cause of hemorrhoids is not as easily traced as that of ulcers. A variety of emotional problems have been identified in individual cases. A professional man who wrote a book and became upset when it did not sell well, developed painful hemorrhoids. A young woman who had trouble getting rid of a boyfriend developed hemorrhoids. In both cases, there was a terminal aspect to the circumstances, – so often the physical punishment fits the emotional crime – but no general statement can be made to pin down the cause of hemorrhoids, other than it, too, is emotionally based, with frustration a prime suspect.

The family doctor used to insist that the ulcer patient take a long trip. He would then get absorbed in his travels and forget his business troubles. But then soon after his return to these same troubles — the same ulcers.

Certain foods are found to be lubricating and coating to the intestinal tract. Carrot juice and okra juice are two of the most common. Often the doctor will restrict these foods from the patient's diet because of the roughage. If the juices of these two particular vegetables are utilized, they could be the most beneficial of all food intake. They are not only lubricating in their action, but the high content of carotene, vitamin A, in carrot juice is essential in the healing process.

Okra with its goodly amount of chlorophyll also promotes more rapid healing in addition to its coating effect and lubricating action. Okra also seems to have a wonderful quality of absorbing the excessive acids and body toxins.

I find it more advisable to eliminate milk, eggs, and any antacid preparations while using carrots and okra for maximum healing and alleviation of the hemorrhoids and ulcers.

To maintain as nearly complete digestion of all food particles which may cause scratching or irritation to the tissues if undigested, it is recommended to use, with meals, two ounces of papaya concentrate which may be diluted with water if desired and bromelain (pineapple enzyme), which may be purchased in health food stores or similar retail stores. As explained earlier in this chapter, these are natural digestive enzymes.

An article in the *American Heart Journal* of April, 1973 pointed out a relationship between varicose veins and hemorrhoids. It hypothesized that because high residue diets promote a more rapid flow of unformed stool compared to low residue diets which require longer transit times and prolonged contact with intestine and colon of hard, rigidly formed stools, the low residue diets promote piles.

This sounds plausible and in the absence of any other causes being identified, I would vote for a diet with adequate bulk as a preventative to hemorrhoids or piles.

I said "preventative." If you have piles, it is like locking the stable door after the horse is stolen. If you have piles, you need to avoid roughage foods.

It is advisable to eliminate scratchy foods, such as coarse

ground cereals, nuts, and whole grain breads in cases of ulcers and hemorrhoids.

I once suffered from hemorrhoids and was told seven years ago by a proctologist after examination, that the fissures would definitely require surgery. However, this condition has been completely alleviated without surgery by using two foods, carrot juice and okra juice, along with papaya concentrate.

A PLANT WITH HEALING POWER YOU CAN GROW AT HOME

There is a greenish-gray cactus that grows naturally in the tropics and subtropics that has been a medical friend to man for centuries. It is called *Aloe Vera,* or true aloe. It is found in abundance in Florida and Hawaii. It is grown everywhere in the United States, usually indoors, as an ornamental plant. Many people do not realize that the plant they have in the windowsill pot can relieve their ulcers or heal a burn.

Alexander the Great knew about aloe, as did the pharaohs of ancient Egypt. In India, China, and Tibet the aloe has been used for centuries for skin conditions and as a laxative.

The ancients split the aloe leaf and spread the raw gel from inside the leaf on skin lesions or burns. The gel has an almost magical effect on burns, preventing blisters and soreness. The Indians in the Florida area have had great respect for the aloe plant and it is part of their fountain of youth legends.

Lately, medical studies have been made on the effects of the aloe plant in healing X-ray burns, and even more recently on radiation burns.

I'll tell you in a forthcoming chapter how to use the aloe for burns, but at this point we are interested in its use for stomach ailments.

The leaves of the aloe are like lances edged with spines. They feel like they are stuffed with sponge rubber. Actually, the stuffing is the gel that you use. Just pull off a mature leaf and squeeze some of the gel into water. Drink the water and almost immediate relief can be felt for stomach irritations and ulcers.

Remember, not all similar cacti are edible. So make sure the plant you use is really the remarkable Aloe Vera.

SOME MODERN MYTHS ABOUT HELPING STOMACH PROBLEMS

When servicemen returned from Vietnam, they were starved for milk and ice cream. They drank and ate it liberally and wondered why they were bloated and gassy. Some had loose acid bowels and others diarrhea.

What was happening was that their digestive system was running short of lactose, the intestinal enzyme that breaks down lactose. Incomplete digestion resulted.

Incomplete digestion causes stomach problems. Milk is one of our excesses. Some doctors think milk should only be consumed by infants and growing children. Some of us do not have the ability to handle a lot of milk. That is why I soft pedal milk in ulcer cases. Many doctors tell their ulcer patients to drink milk to coat their stomach. But why coat the stomach with something that puts a load on the digestive system when it is just as easy to coat the stomach with carrot and okra juice so easily digested.

The greatest modern myth being foisted on the American people is that antacids help your stomach. I have already described how they can be a misnomer in that they can create rather than decrease stomach acid. Now a team of researchers headed by Dr. David Reeder at the Medical Branch of the University of Texas has discovered that calcium carbonate, an ingredient of a score of popularly used antacids, nearly doubles the secretion rate of gastric acid among patients with duodenal ulcer.

What happens is the calcium in calcium carbonate stimulates the production of the hormone gastrin which in turn stimulates the outpouring of acid — exactly what the ulcer sufferer *does not* need.

In closing this chapter on the digestion, let me say a word about another myth. People with stomach problems tend to blame vegetables.

"I should not have eaten the string beans. They're stringy." Or, "I should not have eaten the peas" — for whatever reason.

Others might eat the vegetables, but only providing they are cooked until they are soft.

I say rubbish, and I mean both the idea about vegetables and what you get when you overcook them.

Vegetables are your source of healing. If the old folks could hear me, they would chorus, "Amen." When you are ready to eat following a stomach disorder, eat vegetables.

Now they do not have to be soft. They get soft in your intestional tract. If you cook them soft, the healing power goes into the cooking water.

Steaming is one way to cook vegetables all the way through without pouring most of the vitamins down the drain and injuring the minerals. Steamers can be bought in stores. But you can put a rack on the bottom of any pan that has a tight fitting cover. Put only enough water in so that the surface of the rack is above the water level. Depending on the length of time necessary to cook, you can use less water or may need more water. Thicker cauliflower needs more time to cook, so more water will steam away. String beans cook quickly so less water is needed.

Flavor is retained. Minerals are intact. Vitamins are preserved and ready to do their healing work.

Pass the steamed Brussels sprouts, please.

12

HOW TO HARNESS NATURE TO LIFT YOUR ENERGY LEVELS

The Four Horseman of the Apocalypse, in Revelation of the New Testament, are Fatigue, Old Age, Disease, and Death. Notice that fatigue comes first as a possible precursor of aging.

In this chapter we will examine ways to prevent our energy from being sapped needlessly and ways to build energy from nature's storehouse.

The sun is a source of energy for all life. Even in areas where the sun shines weakly or briefly, its rays are utilized by fauna and flora to survive. Mankind needs sunshine. Some sources say that about ten minutes of direct sunlight on face or hands will satisfy the body's essential need for sun.

The old ways of life required being outdoors for longer periods than today. Ten minutes would be nothing then. Ten minutes in the sun today is for some people a radical adjustment.

I repeat, we need the energy of the sun. Too little is a deprivation, too much is a danger.

WHAT THE SUN CAN DO FOR YOU AND TO YOU

Children need the sun more than adults do. The direct rays of the sun permit them to metabolize vitamin D. When bones have fully matured and reached their normal size, then the sun's rays are no longer required for this particular function.

Some research has been done on natural light versus artificial light. There is increasing evidence that the full spectrum of light is utilized by the body for a number of functions, and indeed may be as important for animals as for plants.

You would not find pre-Edison people lighting candles or lamps in the daytime. Shades were lifted and curtains opened to let in the daylight. Now we just flick a switch. Artificial lights are on during the day almost as much as at night.

Some of the ways we are paying for this, besides the electric bill, are being pointed up by this research. For instance, the fur of animals improves in natural light, bringing up one reason why baldness comes sooner and more frequently to Dad these days than it did to his Dad.

Light passing through the retina affects pineal and pituitary glands, according to these studies, which means the total health is being affected.

A good report on this research is made by Dr. John N. Ott in his book *Health and Light.** He notes how, in Africa, health problems arose when natives began to wear sunglasses, — and nothing else. It is largely the result of the research which he highlights that fluorescent bulb manufacturers and window manufacturers are planning to produce closer to full spectrum products.

Full spectrum means natural. Where have we heard that word before!

But too much of a good thing can be dangerous. Too long in the direct rays of the sun as a daily practice can lead to skin cancer. Certainly it ages the skin, makes it leathery, wrinkled and dry.

How much is too much? It differs with your complexion. Light people can tolerate less. It differs with the season and the time of the day and the latitude. Any exposure which burns you quickly is too much. Gradual tans acquired as a vacation process are fine, but people whose way of life involves long periods in the sun all

*Old Greenwich, Conn.: Devin-Adair Company, Inc., 1974.

year round need to take precautions, especially at mid-day and during spring and summer months.

The farmers still wear Gramps' kind of straw hat. Cowboys have their own wide-brimmed protectors. Women still wear bonnets and bandanas. Women of Japanese origin are seen carrying parasols today on the sidewalks of Honolulu.

The body has to work hard to compensate for the hot rays of excessive amounts of exposure to the sun. In effect, a cooling system has to be turned on. Sweat glands go into operation, often drawing on water supplies needed for other vital purposes. We can become dehydrated.

Little wonder we come in out of the sun feeling exhausted. Exhaustion and sunstroke are the acute effects of too much sun.

Nature's treasure of solar energy needs to be taken in moderation when taken directly. However, you can get many of the benefits of the sun indirectly, through plants and animals.

QUICK ENERGY FOODS THAT FEED YOU, NOT FOOL YOU

If we were to believe everything we read in the ads on the packages, whenever we needed energy we would eat a bowl of sugared flakes or a candy bar or drink a Coke.

These foods do indeed give you a lift.

Then they drop you flat.

You wind up lower than you started out, in no time. Color that whole picture a dismal gray.

There are quick energy foods that do not let you down. And guess who manufactures them — nature.

Grape juice is probably one of the most, if not the most readily assimilated food for quick energy. I have put a number of patients, who were weak and emaciated, on an exclusive grape juice diet. They have reported having more energy on this type of diet than on meat, potatoes, and gravy.

Most fresh fruit and vegetable juices seem to be assimilated quicker raw than if cooked. It is also felt that fruit and vegetable juices can be digested more rapidly than animal protein. The general idea of quick energy foods is how fast these foods can be assimilated by the body. It is found in the average person that certain foods are more compatible with other foods, such as meats with acid foods. Two or more foods that require a longer time and more varied digestive juices for digestion would be heavy starches, such as, pastries, bread, potatoes, corn combined with highly acid foods, such as, tomatoes, peaches, etc. The more the body has to work to digest its source of energy, the less the net energy advantage.

Certain vegetable proteins are easier to digest. For example, green beans are more digestible when compared to navy beans.

Some authorities feel that raw, fresh cabbage juice is another good quick energy food as opposed to cooked cabbage.

One tablespoon of honey in a glassful of warm water may be a good quick energy food in some cases. The bees have already digested honey for you.

A large slug of honey, sometimes up to four ounces, is occasionally used by Olympic athletes to give them the surge of energy they need. But a tablespoonful will do the job for most people.

These two fruit and vegetable juices and natural sweetners like honey or maple syrup contain more than carbohydrate fuel. They contain nutrients and some other hard to identify factor that seems to make nature's products far more energizing than man's.

You might call that factor — life force.

FOODS THAT SAP YOUR ENERGY AND INDUCE FATIGUE

If you were to happen to buy a brand of grape juice — and it is highly unlikely that this would ever happen — which was colored with artificial colorants, preserved with chemicals, and treated with other chemical additives for one reason or another, do you think the grape juice would be as energy giving as natural, untreated grape juice?

Our good sense tells us no. We are giving the body unnatural substances to contend with — either to assimilate, store, or eliminate. More work for the body. Less energy for you.

Testimony before a Senate investigating committee in September, 1972, indicated that many potentially hazardous additives are being used to prolong shelf life with little regard for their possible cumulative effect on people. Furthermore, witnesses pointed out that these additives were not essential to the preservation of that food as they were not used by many competitively priced brands.

There is a new interest in the food industry in imitation foods, like imitation mayonnaise, low cholesterol egg substitutes, and nondairy creamers. Quick energy or question mark?

Your body girds for war whenever foreign elements are introduced. Is there any wonder you occasionally feel depleted, fatigued, weary?

For quick energy, I vote for

Grape Juice

and special mention to

Cabbage Juice
Raw Beet Juice
Honey in Water

ENERGY WITH EVERY BREATH YOU TAKE

For quick energy, I also vote for — oxygen.

Most of us breathe minimally — that is, just enough to keep us alive.

Oxygen is the life-giving — and energy-giving component of our atmosphere. The air we breathe contains about one-fifth oxygen. When life begins to fail, pure oxygen is often given as an emergency measure. By just breathing normally the ailing person can get five times the normal oxygen.

Country folk still take a few deep breaths when they first step out in the fresh morning air. It is invigorating.

The famous physical hygienist Paul Bragg, now 95 years young, teaches what he calls "Super brain breathing" which is basically expanding the diaphragm and stomach area to take in as much "oxygen — the greatest of earthly purifiers" as possible. A few deep breaths, energetically inhaled and energetically exhaled, can give you a feeling of effervescence and youthful enthusiasm.

Yogic breathing is a slower process. Yogis breathe in gently to prolonged counts, hold, and then exhale also slowly and to the same count.

You can do this hatha yoga breathing by sitting on the floor cross-legged, back upright, hands on the knees, eyes straight ahead. Breathe in through your nose to the count of six, each count being about a second. Hold the breath to the count of six. Exhale to the count of six. Do this ten times.

This breathing acts more to step up the metabolism for prolonged energy, whereas the few quick deep breaths provide instant energy.

A walking-breathing activity is often effective in building quick and lasting energy. Here is how it goes:

1. Walk at a normal pace.
2. Inhale, counting as you go.
3. Exhale slowly taking twice the inhalation count.

This is a good way to energize the whole body as oxygen — the cornerstone of life energy — is circulated to the entire body.

It is fun doing this rhythmic breathing while dancing or engaging in some other activity. Waltz or skate and breathe deeply and rhythmically as you move around the floor or over the ice.

HOW TO ENERGIZE COLD, SLUGGISH OR SLEEPY ARMS AND LEGS

Many people find that their arms are weak or their legs fall asleep easily. The blood may have plenty of life energy in it, but it does not seem to be reaching the extremities.

Stiffness, soreness, and coldness to the feet and hands are common complaints. This simple remedy will help to eliminate these conditions by causing a better circulation to these extremities. Do not use when open lesions are present.

Here is what I recommend that you can do *(Figure 12-1)*:

a. Get two pans deep enough to submerge the area to be treated. Four to six inches deep is usually sufficient.
b. Fill one pan with water as hot as possible to the touch. Fill the other pan with cold water (even a few ice cubes will help.)
c. Submerge the area to be stimulated in the cold water for ninety seconds.
d. Remove, and place the area in the very warm water for three minutes.
e. Repeat this procedure twelve times, at least twice daily.

You will notice a remarkable change.

This hot-cold water remedy is a versatile hand-me-down. Take what it did for Mrs. S. and Mrs. A.

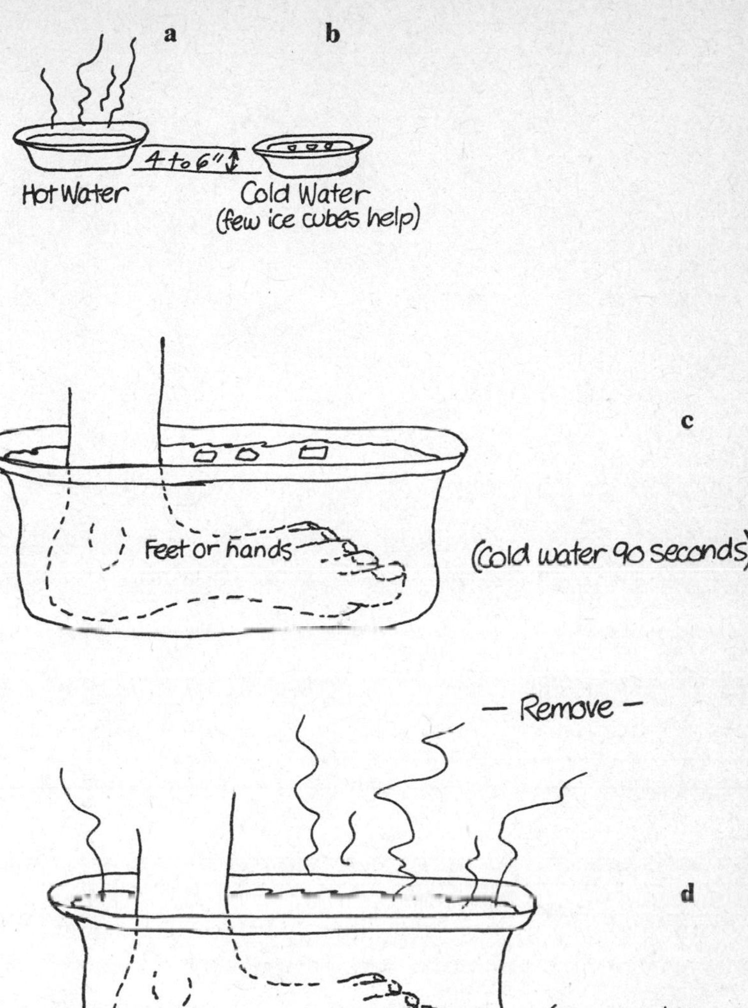

Figure 12-1

Mrs. S. was in her early 80's. She complained to me about her cold feet. She had been wearing bed socks in summer as well as in winter for the past twenty-five years. Her feet were still uncomfortably cold. She was instructed in the use of this hot-cold water therapy. After using it daily, within a week to ten days she was able to eliminate the bed socks. She reported to me how much better she rested at nights because of warmer feet.

Mrs. A., 74 years of age, had a different problem. Her main complaint was stiffness in her wrists from "rheumatiz." I instructed her in the use of this water therapy. She returned to my office three days later very happy with the relief from pain it had given her. She also showed me how much farther she could bend her wrists.

In an earlier chapter on circulation I recommended red beets as a natural remedy. If your lack of energy is evident in your extremities, then beets can help you by helping your circulation.

Mrs. J., a lady in her late 60's, came to my office with the complaint of poor circulation. Her complexion was pale, the whites of her eyes did not have a clear look, and her hands were colder upon touch than they should have been.

She seemed to get a reasonable amount of exercise. Her diet was normally balanced. Upon checking her blood pressure, I found it to be subnormal, but not excessively so. She also had the complaint of feeling tired and lacking in energy. Because she was not lacking in any particular nutrient, I suggested she eat red beets, and drink two ounces of extracted raw beet juice twice a day with morning and evening meals.

Because the lady had traveled a long distance to consult with me, it was approximately one month later before she returned. I was very surprised to see a much more ruddy complexion, with the whites of her eyes clear. The temperature of her hands was warmer and normal; and upon checking her blood pressure, it had improved to within a normal range. This lady told me that her energy was so much greater since using this simple diet.

This gave her the very stimulus she needed. She looked more vital and was able to do a day's work without feeling fatigued.

Many older people used to look at any red foods as energy foods. Today we know that the red color does have an effect on energy levels. But, of all the red foods around, I'll stick to beets as a great circulation and energy source, and I'll point to its natural sugar content as the probable key to its remedial value.

Sometimes the bloodstream should be compensating for special work being done by areas of the body but for some reason is not responding.

For instance, if you work with your hands, they may tire easily or get numb. They are fine at other times but do not rise to the occasion when extra energy is required.

John T. worked as a machinist in a local machine shop. There was a certain amount of physical dexterity required by tightening lathe chisels, with the upper shoulder area involved. However, his work was not so much physical as it was the periodical inspection with calipers of shafts being turned to a certain diameter. John was not a heavily built, muscular man. However, he was developed enough physically for the work he performed. Upon examination, neurologic, orthopedic, and by X-ray, it was determined there was no apparent disability.

He should have been able to perform his work without the discomfort he suffered. I recommended that John take a hot shower, then rub down his arms, neck, and shoulder muscles with common, ordinary vinegar. It should be used full strength and for two or three minutes. Then he was to shower with cold water. This seemed to apparently stimulate the circulation adequately enough to relieve the numbness of his initial complaint.

This remedy goes way back. It combines the hot-cold method with a special stimulating effect of the acetic acid in vinegar.

One cannot complete a list of energy foods without mentioning liver. Calf liver, beef liver, chicken liver — all contain concentrated nutrients. Some people prefer to concentrate these nutrients more by buying desiccated liver. This is liver from which the moisture has been removed. This not only concentrates it in powder form, but preserves it.

Liver is the shot-gun remedy for fatigue. Whatever your body is lacking in the energy department, liver can supply.

Recently, B. H. Ershoff, M.D., did an endurance experiment with rats. He divided them into three groups. Group I was fed a basic, vitamin fortified diet. Group II ate the fortified diet plus extra B complex vitamins. Group III ate the fortified diet plus ten percent dessicated liver added.

Then he placed these groups in separate drums of water from which they could not climb out. Group I and II swam a little over thirteen minutes each before they gave up. Group III swam from one to two hours.

Dessicated liver gave these rats ten times their usual endurance.

If it were not for the poisons used by some meat growers, I would unhesitatingly recommend liver as a regular energy food. Regardless, it is still an energy food with a great big plus.

HOW TO REPAIR THE DRAIN PLUG IN YOUR ENERGY RESERVOIR

"But, doctor," you say, "I eat right and I breathe right, my circulation is fine. I get plenty of sunshine and fresh air. But still I'm fatigued before the day is hardly under way."

"Well," I reply, "You're better off than the person who had both an identity crisis and an energy crisis. He did not know who he was and was too tired to find out."

Seriously, what are you really telling me? You are saying that your energy reservoir is being fed by many sources, but it still never gets really filled.

Maybe the plug is not in the drain.

There are many ways that we permit energy to drain out of us unnecessarily. Standing, walking, sitting, lifting.

When the body is in proper balance, the internal organs have room to function. There is less energy required by them, more energy left over for you.

Foot imbalance is most commonly revealed by an inward roll — too much weight placed on the inner edge of the foot. It can happen to people with high arches as well as those with flat feet. The strain of this imbalance passes up through the knees into the pelvis. It can cause spinal tension which in turn can fatigue you.

Check your stand. Go to where there is some loose sand or sandy soil. Stand barefooted. Examine your footprint. The heel indentation should be nearly equal on both sides, inner and outer of each foot.

If the inner edge is deeper, showing more weight there and an inward roll, you may benefit by doing some simple foot exercises to strengthen all the muscles in your feet and discourage your favoring one part of your foot.

Stand barefoot on a thick board, or a cinder block, or even a large thick book. Curl your toes down around the front edge, keeping your balance on the balls of your feet.

Here is another good foot movement. Again barefoot, raise yourself on your toes. Hold for five seconds and then lower your heels again to the normal standing position. Repeat ten times.

Here's one you can do while sitting down anywhere. You need to take your shoes off, though. Place feet flat on the floor. Raise toes up. Spread toes apart. Hold toes apart a few seconds. Now squeeze them together. You can repeat this a few times, one foot at a time or both feet together *(Figure 12-2).*

Standing stoop-shouldered is another great energy-draining error. It is a tough habit to break. But once you discover how you look by seeing your profile in a full length mirror, you will want to consciously stand erect until this becomes a new habit. With

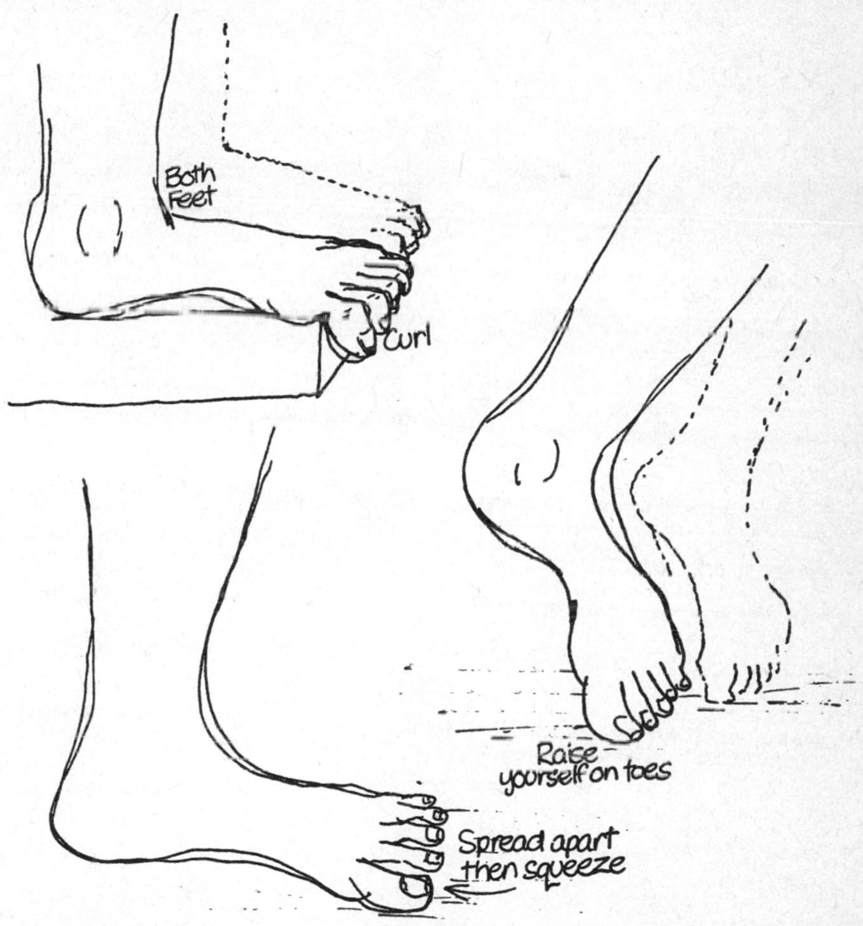

Figure 12-2

Foot Movements

your back in proper alignment, it takes less of an expenditure in energy to carry your body weight. This leaves more energy for you to carry out your day's work.

To correct your posture, you need to know the feel of good posture. Start the day off reminding yourself of this feeling. Here is how:

Upon arising in the morning, stand back to a wall. Now make sure the following parts of your body are touching the wall. Check each out in turn — heels...calves...thighs...buttocks...shoulders...back of head. Now walk away from the wall, holding this posture and memorizing the feeling.

You must plug up the energy drain in walking.

First, refresh your memory of that back-to-wall posture. Then, as you take your first step, let the whole body incline slightly forward. Remember, there is no bending from the waist. The whole body inclines from the bottom of the feet to the top of the head. Arms hang freely at the sides, swinging in a natural response to the gait.

Again, it is difficult to acquire a correction immediately in something we do unconsciously or automatically for a long period of time. But, with repetition of the full body incline, a new walking habit can be acquired, one which will save you many foot-pounds of work every day.

THE ENERGY-SAVING WAY TO LIFT

No matter whether we are in the house all day, behind a desk, or in a warehouse, lifting is an activity that we find ourselves involved in constantly.

Lifting improperly can tire us. Lifting in the correct way can be practically effortless.

If we take more energy to lift than the proper way dictates, then we are also risking eventual injury.

During my 25 years in practice I have treated hundreds of men and women who have come to me with back problems and injuries caused more by improper lifting than by over-lifting.

The most common type of improper lifting occurs when a person bends over straight-legged (without bending the knees) and attempts to lift some object, thereby inviting severe pain to the back.

I have instructed these people in the correct way to lift. I have talked with them two or three years later and found that they have been able to do their work without the previous discomfort suffered merely by taking these precautions in their lifting. I feel that most doctors could better help their patients who have so-called back strains by finding out how the patient acquired the injury and cautioning him against further injury by improper bending while lifting.

Here are some helpful hints for proper lifting:

1. Always keep the back straight when lifting.
2. Squat down within easy reach of the object to be lifted.
3. Keep the arms and the object being lifted close to the body.
4. Let the leg and arm muscles do the work of lifting.
5. Lift only objects within the size and weight of your strength — *Know your strength.*

HOW YOUR CAR CAN DRAIN YOUR ENERGY AND WHAT TO DO ABOUT IT

When your car gives you a lift, you may think you are saving your energy, but I have found that the simple act of driving to and from work can tax a person's energy more than walking, depending on two factors:

1. Stress
2. Posture

When you leave your quiet living room and a few minutes later are moving swiftly along a highway or freeway, you have moved from a tranquil environment to an environment fraught with tension and anxiety. Every minute involves decision-making again and again. Every decision involves mental stress and strain which consumes energy and every mental stress and strain creates its counterpart in the physical body which in turn wastes more energy.

Relaxing while driving under present day traffic conditions is well nigh to impossible. It is easier to relax driving fifty miles an hour on a freeway than thirty miles an hour on urban or suburban streets.

If we approach each driving event in a relaxed way, we emerge from it more relaxed than if we started off tense.

So car energy saver number one is begin your drive confidently and serenely.

When you are under way, you can save energy by being alert mentally rather than physically. If you watch some people when they drive, they are like a batter stepping up to the plate. They wrap themselves around the steering wheel and tense their legs up at the gas and brake pedals as if that made them readier for some eventuality. When you are hunched over the steering wheel, you are causing hypertension of the neck which in turn creates pressure on spinal nerves in the lower neck and upper back. This translates into — energy drain.

Body tenseness does not make your reflexes any faster. In fact, body tenseness can slow them up. Body tenseness can also interfere with the accuracy of the action or reaction. We tend to *over*-act or *over*-react.

Car energy saver number two is pay attention to your driving. Substitute mental alertness for physical alertness. Whenever your mind makes a decision, your body will carry it out. Physical tenseness might be defined as "you getting in your own way."

Finally, car energy saver number three is to adjust your seat so it is proper for you. A family with many drivers should buy their next car with power seats so each driver can easily adjust the seat to optimum position. You should be able to see over the hood without craning your neck, yet not have to slouch to avoid the ceiling.

I am treating this subject of car travel from an energy level point of view, so daily short trips are the focus. Longer trips require attention to possible back problems which I won't go in to, except to say, get out and stretch frequently. Other aspects of a car that involve our back rather than energy levels are the two-door versus four-door models and how that can induce back strain getting in and out. Also, arm rests, chair tilt, and similar matters come into play.

No wonder, when the first cars came out it was our grandparents' opinion that the most important part was "the nut that holds the steering wheel."

A SIMPLE THERAPY TO BUILD BODY STRENGTH

If you have access to heavy gravel (approximately the size of a hen's egg), which is not imbedded in the yard or driveway, walk barefooted on these rocks if you want a new feeling of vim, vigor, and vitality. Take it rather easy as you will find that you will not be able to stand on these rocks very long the first few times. Try to increase the time of walking gradually.

I have literally seen people pulled out of the grave by using this type of therapy. I treated a man in his seventies, who for years had been having a case of chronic diarrhea. His health was so poor that he had not been able to do any work at all. He did not feel safe to attempt to drive his car.

After daily walks on these rocks for a period of thirty days, he did not appear to be the same individual. For the first time in years he had a healthy color to his face, his eyes sparkled, and he told me he felt that it was worth several thousand dollars to know of this ridiculously simple, yet effective, method of treatment.

If you ask me for a logical medical reason why this works, you won't get it. All I can say is, nature figured man might take millennia to discover beet juice, etc. So nature gave man an automatic energy stimulator, activated when he uses energy in a natural way by walking.

Do I believe nature can demonstrate this much wisdom?

Naturally.

13

SIMPLE WAYS TO HELP YOURSELF TO A LONGER LIFE

There is an old saying that goes: "There is no right way to do a wrong thing."

Irwin Ross, freelance writer, once wrote a humorous item for the Minneapolis *Tribune* in which he told how he used to be treated for a cold as a child by his mother with mounds of blankets, tar and mothballs, whiskey, onion juice, sulfur, and paregoric. He was covered with mustard plasters and given onion soup and tea.

Now, writes Ross good humoredly, he has tried the newest cold tablets. They led to sleepiness, so he got pills from his doctor to combat that. They kept him awake all night, so he took sleeping pills. He broke out in a rash and had to take a drug. That cured the rash but he got stomach cramps. A new medicine helped that, but suddenly changed his sex. After getting bald, growing green mold on his skin, getting convulsions, and other problems, Ross goes back to the blankets and mustard plaster.

We sometimes need an exaggeration like this to begin to see an underlying truth. There is no right way to do a wrong thing.

If we try to correct the situation by doing another wrong thing, we only make matters worse.

Making matters worse may not grow green mold on your skin. It may just take years off your life.

There is no way to eat the wrong foods the right way.

There is no way to place continuous stresses and strains upon the body and expect to adjust to them or correct for them.

Adjustments and corrections remind me of the little boy playing in the sand by the ocean's edge. He builds a sand wall that stops the fingers of water. As the tide comes in, he repairs the eroding sand on his wall. Faster and faster, harder and harder he works, but to no avail. Soon, the water has engulfed his barricade.

If you live your life in a way that exposes you to an erosion or sapping of your strength and vitality, there is no pill that we know about, no operation that will undo the effects.

You must take your medicine — but not the kind that comes in bottles.

THE SINGLE IDEA THAT CAN ADD YEARS TO YOUR LIFE

It was recently pointed out that there are surgeons who will not operate if the patient is convinced he will not survive the operation, even if all other vital signs are "go". Experience has shown that the state of mind is a key vital sign.

You will hear smokers say, "I like smoking. When my time is up, I'll go."

This sounds almost like a death wish.

It is the same with liquor, soda, candy. Let's live for the moment you say, "I have to die sometime."

Sorry, you cannot be my patient.

To be my patient you have to want to live. And the longer you want to live the more enthusiastic I become about helping you.

This is the single idea that can add years to your life — the will to live.

"Of course, I want to live," you say. But you need to say it when you reach for a cigarette or a sweet. Otherwise, when you put either in your mouth, you are paying lip service to the idea of a longer life and paying service to your senses instead.

In our society we are trained to grow old and die. It starts at youth. We are told to respect our old and feeble grandparents.

We see our parents age. We are sold life insurance and learn the age at which we are "expected" to die according to the life expectancy tables.

Social pressures and cultural norms work on us so that by the time we reach the fifties and sixties we begin to manifest the same aging characteristics that others have before us. Then we "obey" the actuarial table.

I see more and more statements from educators and scientists that call our attention to this error in our beliefs. They point out:

- The aging process can be slowed down.
- There is no reason why people should be dying at the present actuarial ages.
- A person who expects to become helpless at 85 or 90 is helping to bring that about.
- Senility is not a required condition in aging.
- There is no principle in nature that prevents our living much longer life spans in optimum health.

Barring accident, murder, or suicide, there is never any one cause of death. It is a lot of little contributing factors that add up. Then something starts to give.

In this chapter I am going to assume you are not interested in committing slow suicide and that you want to live a longer, healthier life.

FIRST AID – PRACTICING SELF CARE EFFECTIVELY

If we could flash back to earlier days, we would get the impression that the old-fashioned mother fussed too much. She would treat the least mishap as a crisis. On would go the water to boil, or out would come the hot packs or cold packs.

Today, we tend to ignore a swelling, a cut, or a bruise. A slight sprain is no reason to stay off an ankle, so we walk on it. Maybe there is no observable aftereffect and we say triumphantly, "See?" But aftereffects may not be observable. It might be that the healing did not take place as efficiently as it would have had we given nature full rein and stayed off the ankle. Years later we might have to pay for this.

A devil-may-care attitude about slight injuries is similar to the attitude that a little poison won't hurt. Practice self-care every minute of your life and you will add years to that statistical life expectancy.

Self-care starts with first aid. Here are some tried and true ways to take care of minor injuries until a doctor can be consulted.

Swelling. Talking only about the extremities — swelling in the wrist, knee, finger, toe, elbow, ankle, etc. — is your body's way of protecting the area. It insulates the bruise so healing can take place and further injury prevented. Ice packs can relieve swelling to the extent that they change circulation in the area. It is wise after applying ice packs to have your doctor check for possible dislocations, fracture, or ruptured blood vessels.

Throbbing. Sometimes pain and throbbing follow a knock or bump. Again, an ice pack can relieve this symptom. The pounding with each heart beat is frequently felt in the head and mistaken for simple headache.

Mrs. Alice D. had been having recurring throbbing (pounding with each heartbeat) headaches for years, which had incapacitated her from doing her housework. Sedation was ineffective. Her condition had been previously diagnosed by her doctor as migraine due to an imbalance of circulation to the brain.

She was instructed to go home upon leaving my office and lie down in her bed with her feet on ice packs, no pillow under head, but to remain comfortable and warm under blankets if necessary. She later reported after fifteen minutes of this procedure the pounding in her head subsided. She was instructed to use this procedure again if it ever returned.

Nosebleeds. Normal nosebleeds are the ones we are talking about here. These are the ones resulting from a sharp blow to the nose, too much or too hard blowing of the nose, or scratching the interior of the nostril with the finger or other object. If not brought on by any of these factors, see your doctor as a nosebleed, especially repeated or persistent, can be a symptom of some other disorder.

However, normal nosebleeds can be treated by having the person sit still. Do not lie down as this increases blood pressure in the head. Sitting still alone may do the trick. If the bleeding seems to be from the soft, lower part of the nose, pinch the nostrils together and hold this way a few minutes. You can use a clothespin or the fingers. Release carefully so as not to disturb the coagulation that has formed. If from the upper part of the nose, out of reach of such pressure, apply a cold compress on the nose. Another cold compress on the back of the neck may also help. These ice packs cause reflex constriction of the blood vessels and encourage sealing of the opening. After the bleeding stops, the nose should not be blown for as long as possible so as not to disturb the protective clotting that has formed. If bleeding has not stopped in five or ten minutes, a doctor should be consulted.

Burns. Most burns are classified as first, second, or third degree. First degree burns cause a redness of the skin. Second degree burns cause blistering. Third degree burns cause a damaging, like charring, of the tissue. These third degree burns should be treated by a doctor. First and second degree burns can be treated at home. In a previous chapter I mentioned the aloe plant. If you have one growing, break off the top of a leaf, squeeze some sap out on the burn, and that will probably be the end of your pain or soreness. If no aloe, try ice. Ice restricts the blood vessels and cuts down on later blisters and swelling.

Cuts. Again, we are not talking about the gaping wound that needs a doctor to stitch it, but shallow cuts. Wash gently with soap. Cleanliness is the important goal. Once free of foreign matter, bind the cut with a sterile bandage.

First aid in accidents is another matter. Many injuries can result from everyday chores, in and out of the home — near drownings, broken bones, third degree burns. Your local Red Cross, and possibly your local police, have illustrated literature explaining just what to do until medical care arrives.

The old washtubs may not have been as efficient as modern bathtubs and showers but they were a lot safer. Accidents that take place in bathtubs and showers today cost Americans over 70 million dollars a year in medical costs, thirty percent happening with children under five. Provide bath seats for children. Install secure hand holds with rounded edges for adults.

Take care. But if something accidental happens to you, be sure it is taken care of.

WHAT TO DO ABOUT STUBBORN SORES AND HARD TO HEAL LESIONS

Mrs. Anna G., 70 years of age, had a sore one-fourth inch in diameter on the side of her face for six months before she came to me. It had been diagnosed as non-malignant. All ointments had failed to heal it. I recommended to this lady, as a home treatment, to keep a constant application of a gauze pad saturated with pure Concord (purple) grape juice, undiluted. She was instructed not to scrub or wash off the sore area. Within three weeks, the sore had healed completely. There was a very minimum scar tissue visible.

Another case was that of a registered nurse, Mrs. Gertrude A., age 40, who had a necrotic sore on the posterior section of her heel, three-eights inch in diameter, with a depth opening showing the bone. The condition had persisted for fourteen years. It had not grown any larger or smaller during this period of time. It had resisted all medication and therapies, including cobalt radiation.

This patient was instructed to soak her heel in a crockery container (*no metal)* filled with adequate Concord grape juice before bedtime for thirty minutes daily. After soaking her heel, she was directed to very gently pat the sore area dry with cotton, but not to wash or get the area wet while bathing.

In two weeks, Mrs. A. returned to my office. The lesion was more than three-fourths healed. One week later she again returned, and the lesion was completely healed with no scab and a smooth surface of skin. Needless to say, she was very amazed with the healing quality of the grape juice.

What is there about grape juice that gives it this healing quality? Nature knows. My own theory is that Concord grape juice contains potassium, phosphorus, and some calcium — in usable and balanced form proportions. It also has a high astringent quality.

It has even helped with the tiny cuts and abrasions caused by athlete's foot. Don't sell grape juice short, just because it is a drink and not like a medicine or antiseptic. Nature does not reveal all her secrets. But they work.

Well, enough about injuries and first aid. Let's talk about staying well, maintaining resistance to disease, and living longer.

BREAD THE OLD WAY IS REALLY THE STAFF OF LIFE

There has been a lot said about "empty calories" in recent years. Much of this has been directed at refined and sugared cereals. Also deserving of this label is refined white bread.

Even when the label says "fortified" or "enriched," what has been put back into the bread is in no way equal to what was taken out in the refining process.

The way flour used to be ground and the way bread used to be baked made bread a food, in fact a valuable food, worthy of the title "staff of life."

The way bread is made now, it is usually more harm to us than good, especially if eaten in large quantities.

Most of us eat bread every day. Even if we eat just two pieces of toast in the morning and no more bread the rest of the day, we consume some three thousand loaves of bread in a lifetime.

There is just a little chemical preservative in a loaf of bread, and a little freshener, and a little of perhaps another chemical or two. But multiply that by three thousand and you are asking your body to find a way to get rid of a quantity of mild poison greater than your own weight.

A few pieces of white bread place a stress on your body that you can measure:

Take your pulse before breakfast, or any other meal in which you eat bread or rolls. Then take it again about a half hour later. Your pulse will rise as the body labors to get rid of what we call the staff of life.

Some staff. More like a club that we keep hitting our body with every single day.

In his book *The Doctor's Proven New Home Cure For Arthritis,** Dr. Giraud Çampbell tells how he has cured hundreds of people suffering from arthritis, many of whom had been bedridden for years. It is done largely through diet and Dr. Campbell points the finger of guilt at processed foods in general and bread in particular. To keep free of arthritis, his cured patients must keep free of bread.

---

*West Nyack, N.Y.: Parker Publishing Company, Inc., 1972.

Other diseases are adversely affected by refined flour, like kidney problems, hardening of the arteries, and sinus.

It was not always thus. There was a time when bread was indeed the staff of life. This was when it was made from stone ground whole grains. The whole grain contains protein, the body builder. It contains iron and other minerals to build blood: soothe nerves, and regulate your body. Vitamins B_1 and B_2 contribute to clear vision and healthy skin. Niacin helps your body extract nutrients from the other foods you eat.

All this is in the bread Grandma used to bake.

She used additives, too. But natural additives, like brewer's yeast which helps to complete the protein and add more B-complex vitamins.

If you bake bread, use whole wheat flour. You can obtain it at health food stores. Consider your own natural additives like

- Kelp. Iodine-rich and better than salt.
- Soy flour. Adds more protein.
- Wheat germ. Here are the B- vitamins extracted from other bread.
- Bran. A mineral-rich roughage.
- Bone meal powder. High in calcium.

STAY AWAY FROM THESE PEOPLE IF YOU WANT TO LIVE LONGER

Smokers need not read this section because I am talking about you and you cannot really stay away from yourself. If you have not heeded the words of the Surgeon General of the United States on every package of cigarettes, then my words would probably go unheeded, too.

You non-smokers are not as safe from the life-shortening effects of tobacco smoke as you may think.

In a recent statement (November, 1975) pointing out the continued increase in cancer mortality in countries where smoking is widespread, The World Health Organization also stated, "The non-smoker exposed to the side-stream smoke of smokers in enclosed ill-ventilated spaces, such as cars and small offices, may be exposed to harmful concentrations of smoke."

Whereas a decade ago, efforts to legislate bans against smoking in public places may have been considered a joke, today such legislation is on the increase. More and more, people are beginning to exercise their right to breath air unfouled by tobacco smoke. Measures restricting smoking in public places have been enacted in some thirty states.

For instance, Minnesota has banned smoking in almost any public place except where designated smoking areas are set up, and my state, Kansas, has enacted a law against smoking on any premises where the person in charge posts no-smoking signs.

An organization known as Group Against Smokers' Pollution (GASP) is in the process of educating people on the serious implications of breathing secondhand smoke. A list of the nearly fifty poisons in tobacco smoke sounds like an inventory for chemical warfare. These include pyridine, furfural, acrolein, hydrocyanic acid, hydrogen cyanide, and worse.

Some of the most hazardous compounds are in greater concentrations in the sidestream smoke — that is, the smoke from the burning end — than in the mainstream smoke inhaled by the smoker. There is twice as much tar and nicotine in the sidestream smoke; three times as much benzpyrene, suspected as a cancer causing agent, and fifty times as much ammonia.

Carbon monoxide, which robs the blood of oxygen, is a special threat. The Federal Air Quality Standards for outside air is nine parts per million. Yet studies have shown that smoking as few as seven cigarettes by smokers even in a ventilated room can create carbon monoxide levels of twenty p.p.m. and in the seat next to the smoker as high as 90 p.p.m.

Cadmium is another smoker's threat to non-smokers. It is found in concentrated amounts in the lungs, liver, and kidneys where autopsies are performed on emphysema victims. Yet there is even more cadmium that drifts from the burning end of the cigarette.

What good is it if you eat whole grain bread with one hand and poison yourself with the other?

We poison ourselves in many ways. Sometimes they are not that well recognized or as easy to control as tobacco smoke. Take our cooking utensils.

Copper pots and pans are now acknowledged to be harmful and almost all copper cookware is tin-lined. However, aluminum is still being used and it gets into the food you cook in aluminum pots. Figures developed in 1940 and later reprinted in the *Journal of the American Institute of Homeopathy* show that some foods, like creamed cabbage and lemon pie filling with less than one part per million of aluminum naturally, wind up with about one hundred parts per million of aluminum after being cooked in aluminum pots.

What remains controversial is whether aluminum in these quantities is harmful. It certainly is not helpful or nature would place these levels of aluminum in our food, naturally.

Tobacco smoke also had to win this battle of being recognized as harmful. Now that this label of poison has been firmly affixed, avoid smoking — your own or someone else's smoke.

AN EASY WAY TO RELIEVE CONSTIPATION

The body's intake must be pure and the body's elimination of wastes must be efficient. These two factors alone can prolong life.

Some people move their bowels every day, but the wastes that they eliminate might still be a day or two behind schedule. Carrying waste material unnecessarily long periods of time is a burden on the body as they can be reabsorbed by tissues.

Certain foods like beets and corn will show in your stool. They provide a simple test to see whether your bowel movements are on schedule. The red coloring or undigested kernels should show in less than twenty-four hours.

Constipation makes itself known. You miss bowel movements for a day or more.

There is a simple way to accelerate elimination by sluggish organs of elimination. I have found drinking more water can relieve many cases of constipation.

Drink two or three large glasses of cool water rapidly every morning, preferably soon after arising. The cool water is more stimulating to sluggish elimination than warm or tepid water. But do not drink it iced.

Also one should always remember to drink a sufficient quantity of liquids during the day — at least six glasses, taking care not to "wash down" food, thereby diluting the digestive juices which could cause a possible digestive disturbance.

One case I recall is that of Mrs. Beulah H., age 45, housewife, who came to my office with painful low-back condition. After a few treatments, she had made a favorable response, but she seemed to be at a standstill so far as progressing further.

She asked me if constipation could have anything to do with her condition. She had been constipated for a number of years. I explained to her that the constipation which was a secondary symptom to her low-back problem, could be a contributing factor. She was advised to drink three glasses of cool tap water each morning twenty minutes before breakfast.

She made the comment that she didn't feel she could drink that much water. I explained to her that the three glasses of water would tend to flush her system more thoroughly than just two glasses of water would. She consented to try it.

At the next appointment she came in very highly elated to report that she had a thorough, natural bowel movement each morning after using this simple recommendation. Her back condition improved much more rapidly, and within two weeks of time she was pain-free.

THE ONE VITAMIN YOUR BODY NEEDS EVERY DAY AND HOW TO KEEP AN INEXPENSIVE NATURAL SUPPLY

If your body is deprived of oxygen, you do not last very many minutes. The next most important requirement is water. Here survival is measured in days. You can go weeks without any food at all.

However, when you are getting your oxygen, water, and food, there is still something you need daily, found in food, but sometimes absent. Its absence can lead to extreme weakness, bleeding, and ultimate death through a disease known as scurvy.

Until the eighteenth century, scurvy was the sailors' nemesis. A few weeks out of port and scurvy inevitably struck. Those members of the crew it did not kill it left in such weakened condition that they were useless — the ship had to head for port. Once there, fresh food brought about recovery. Loosened teeth, black and blue bruises, weakened bones were restored to normalcy.

Captain James Cook (1728-1779) solved the problem. He was no scientist or physician, but he saw the recovery brought about when fresh provisions were taken aboard, especially fruits and vegetables. On one of his voyages he took along barrels of concentrated vegetable soup and additional barrels of sauerkraut. No more scurvy.

What did these vegetables have that was absent from salted meat, salted fish, dried peas, oatmeal, and biscuits? Vitamin C.

People with a vitamin C deficiency look old, feel old, and are indeed old. Actually this deficiency can occur on a daily basis, but of course a day's deficiency is not as pronounced or visible as a month's. Still, it takes its toll in lowered levels of vitality and strength and opens the way to more serious disease by lowering the body's resistance.

Today with frozen vegetables and fruit juices available the year round and good transportation facilities to bring in citrus fruits from the South and other produce from warmer climates, there is no reason to be without vitamin C foods a single day.

Nobel prize winner Dr. Linus Pauling singles out sauerkraut as a good source of vitamin C. Raw sauerkraut is recommended by nutritionists.

In the old days sauerkraut was made in large five gallon crocks. Salted layers of raw shredded cabbage were placed in the earthenware containers and stored in a warm place for about six weeks. Some of the old recipes called for other flavorings to be added to the salt like caraway or mustard seeds, juniper berries or sliced apples.

Today, sauerkraut is easily obtained in the supermarket or smaller grocery stores. Keep it on hand as a reminder that something with vitamin C is in it and is needed by your body every day.

TEN COMMANDMENTS FOR A LONGER LIFE

Dr. Linus Pauling also recommends vitamin E as a life prolonger. He states that this vitamin and vitamin C act as antioxidants destroying free radicals in the tissues which he says contribute to aging.

Certainly if we were to set up some principles to follow in extending one's span of vitality and productive life, these two vitamins as well as others would be included.

Vitamin E is found in navy beans, peas, parsley, and kale. But it is in greater concentrations in wheat germ, wheat germ oil, and soybean oil.

It is not so easy, even for a doctor, to establish principles for longer life. Just when you think you have locked in to one or two, along comes some centenarian who breaks these rules successfully.

Dr. Pauling would have us consume adequate vitamins and minerals, cut down on sugar, avoid tobacco. These principles are certainly hard to argue with.

A recent survey conducted by researchers at the University of California at Los Angeles found that poor health habits were more related to mortality than was income. Some seven thousand Californians were included in the survey, — all age brackets, income brackets, and walks of life.

It was found that those who followed certain good health practices had a level of health equal to those twenty years younger who practiced only a few and ignored the others. No smoking and moderate alcohol were, of course, two. Others were plenty of sleep, good breakfast, no snacks, proper weight, and moderate exercise.

But let me give you my own priorities for a longer, active life. Let's call them the ten commandments for longer, livelier living:

1. Get seven to eight hours of sleep nightly.
2. Eat three well-balanced meals a day.
3. Include bulk foods and mineral and vitamin-rich foods in daily menus.
4. Cut down on sugary foods and chemically-treated foods.
5. Get some fresh air and sunshine every day, if possible.
6. Drink a few glasses of pure, fresh water every day.
7. Do not smoke; stay away from people who do.
8. Avoid alcoholic drinks, except rarely, and then in moderation.
9. Exercise naturally every day, like walking, swimming, or gardening.
10. Use laughter to banish anxiety and fear; let every day be joyous.

14

NATURE'S MARVELOUS HEALTH BOOSTERS

Astronomers have recently discovered that the vast reaches of space are filled with a complex organic molecule capable of forming life.

Previously thought to exist only on earth, methenamine has been detected by radio telescopes throughout our galaxy and as far as these telescopes' range can penetrate — trillions of miles into space. The conclusion is inescapable: life must have formed on other planets as it has on earth.

In fact, the discovery seems to underline the possibility that the universe exists as a vehicle for life to express.

I mention this at the risk of getting overly philosophical in order to point up the power of nature to accomplish her purpose.

And her purpose is your good health.

Why then is good health so hard to maintain? Because we interfere with nature.

There are three major areas where we interfere with nature:

1. We tamper with nature's foods.

2. We substitute energy-saving devices for natural movement.
3. We replace the peacefulness of nature with fear, tenseness, and anxiety.

I am going to end this book with a burst of marvelous remedies and tonics that nature places at our disposal to maintain a high level of vibrant health. But to what avail are they, if we promote good health with one hand while interfering with good health with the other hand.

So before I give you these remedies, I want to remind you of the kind of interference you are running, so you can get out of your own way.

THE MYTH THAT ROUGHAGE IRRITATES THE STOMACH LINING

Elsie R., a widow, came to me with a stomach problem. Solid foods caused indigestion. So she had been sticking to foods that were "slippery and soft" – like cooked cereal, milk, custard, ice cream, white bread.

When I recommended some roughage foods to stimulate the muscular type of action necessary to smooth-functioning digestion, she threw up her hands.

"Oh, no, doctor," she exclaimed in horror, "I would get deathly sick. "Whole-wheat bread? Spinach? Cabbage? Carrots? Those are the kinds of rough foods that irritate my sensitive stomach."

I could tell from the tone of her voice that no amount of explanation by me would upset the conviction that she had. Then I remembered Arthur B., a widower. I got him on the phone.

"I have a patient here with the same stomach problem you used to have. I realize this is an unusual procedure, but if you would be willing to tell her on the phone of your experience in getting rid of it, you would be doing your good turn for the day."

He agreed. I introduced them over the phone. They talked. She got more and more interested. Asked if they could have tea together, so she could get more details. A week later she was back in my office, telling me what a nice man Arthur B. was, sharing with me her late mother's recipe for German coleslaw, and — incidentally — saying how much better she was feeling.

Moral: Sometimes a widower is more convincing than a married doctor, at least to a widow.

Nature offers her way. But we want to superimpose our way. It's not that we are ornery. We just think we know better. Or we let our senses get in the way of sense.

If something manufactured tastes sweeter or smoother, we let its taste get to us, and we let the good sense to avoid its sterility slip away from us.

Smooth and sweet in processed food means sallow and sickly. Smooth means less nutrients absorbed. Sweet, even without being sickly sweet, leeches the body of what little nutrients are available. Crisp and crunchy in natural food, maybe less sensuous to the senses, but it makes better sense to the body.

Soon, as a higher level of health is restored, the sweet tastes of yesterday can no longer be tolerated. Sweet tastes sickly sweet and the sweet tooth becomes a vestigial organ.

Also, crispness and crunchiness, as found in raw or slightly cooked compared to overcooked vegetables, becomes a criterion for good taste.

You can begin this transformation now by substituting fact for myth.

The coarse leaves of lettuce and cabbage and the fibrous material of beets and turnips do not act as crude irritants to the sensitive and delicate lining of the stomach.

Yes, your stomach lining is sensitive and delicate. It is largely mucous membrane, the same as your nostrils, mouth, and throat. However, in the stomach, these cells and tissues are muscular in nature. They need to be stimulated in their digestive action. They also need to be themselves fed in order to perform their digestive action which includes muscular-type movements such as squeezing and grinding.

When smooth food tiptoes by, this digestive stimulation is not activated. And the body, including the digestive system, is starved for nutrition.

Nature is foiled again.

When you get into nature's way, you get into your own way. Eat a variety of natural foods as close to the way nature prepares them as possible and you are giving nature a chance to work for your optimum health.

"DON'T PANIC – WE'RE GOING ORGANIC"

That is the good humored battle cry of health food enthusiasts whose numbers are growing all over the country. Purchases of organic foods have multiplied five fold in the past five years.

Little Miss Muffet would have plenty of company around her tuffet today to enjoy her curds and whey, which translated today reads clabbered milk or more specifically buttermilk, yogurt, or acidophilus milk.

There are now some five thousand health food stores throughout the country and more opening every day specializing in the foods of grandmother's day.

Technically speaking, organic foods are those grown in soil that is organically fertilized, as opposed to commercial fertilizers, artificially or chemically prepared. Organic foods are those grown without the use of chemical pesticides.

These two qualifications must be present for a food to be accurately designated as organic, but unfortunately one or the other is frequently missing in such designated foods.

Supermarkets are now adding health food departments or shelves stocked with the most popular health food products like milled whole grains, seeds, nuts, sun-dried fruits, honey, molasses, and yogurt.

Health food stores go much further depending on what local organic producers are able to supply, like goat's milk, fertile eggs, organically grown meat and vegetables, unprocessed cheese, etc. You can get several kinds of sprouts, seaweed, fresh bread made from a variety of whole grains, and a number of bottled fruit juices and vegetable juices.

Some people go organic because of the growing awareness of possible harmful long term effects of chemical additives and pesticides. Others buy organic foods because they taste better.

The organic trend is not limited to foods. You now see organic shampoos, cosmetics, and toothpastes. Cleaning compounds are made with organic ingredients and soaps are biodegradable. One commercial for a deodorant bragged that its can was "not aerosol." Quite a switch from a few years ago when the wind blew in the other direction.

Observed, each one of these fifteen principles will contribute to a high efficiency of digestion and every cell in your body will say, "Thank you."

THE BEST WAYS TO GET ESSENTIAL PROTEIN

Your body is mostly protein — skin, hair, flesh, muscles, blood, nails, organs, glands, veins, and arteries.

Your body cannot make protein out of other types of food.

These two facts point to one of the most important dietary truths: you must supply your body with essential protein.

Jerome C. came to me complaining of chronic fatigue. His list of complaints was endless. It was like an organ recital.

I could see a lackluster in him. He was a little overweight, but still his body was undernourished.

"You need to eat more protein," I remarked as I was examining him.

"I am a vegetarian, but I eat lots of lentils," he said, "also corn. I looked them up. Both have protein."

"They are not complete protein," I informed him. "And unless you eat the parts that are missing at the same time, it is just like eating no protein at all."

I instructed Jerome to eat corn the same time as beans. Each had what the other was missing. Peanut butter has missing amino acids which make it useless as a protein unless eaten with bread. And I told him about soy beans — a complete protein.

In two weeks Jerome C. was a different man. His step was brisker; his voice was more resonant; and he looked more ruggedly masculine.

Protein comes from a Greek word meaning "first in importance." If it is in short supply, your body "eats" its own muscles in order to keep vital organs going.

It is a complex food, composed of some twenty-two amino acids. Many of these amino acids can be made by the body. But the ones that cannot be made by the body — the so-called essential amino acids — must be eaten in sufficient quantity if protein is to be supplied to the body.

It is like a jig-saw puzzle, especially for vegetarians. You must fit in the missing amino acids when you plan a menu. For meat eaters, every meat, fish, and poultry is a complete protein. So are eggs and cheeses. There are also substantial amounts of complete protein in milk and nuts.

Here are some more "mix and match" tips for vegetarians:

- Mix nuts (brazil) or seeds (sesame) with vegetables.
- Mix red beans with rice.
- Mix grains and cereals with peas, lentils, and beans.

Soybeans are the vegetarian's answer to a protein prayer. The soybean has been called the oldest food crop in the world, still its true value nutritionally has only been fully recognized in the Western world in this century.

Of course, there is resistance from manufacturers of processed foods and cosmetics. And the debate will probably go on for years. But is there any doubt which side of the fence I stand on? — nature's side.

SOME TRIED AND TRUE RULES FOR BETTER DIGESTION

A friend of mine chews his milk.

Another person I know won't eat watermelon for dessert, but will eat it at the start of a meal.

There's a neighbor of mine who won't drink stale coffee that has been standing on the stove a few hours.

People have their pet rules to follow. There must be a thousand of these rules, should anyone ever want to collect them. And you know what? There's some truth in all of them.

The fellow that chews his milk is beginning the digestion of its carbohydrates and preventing the formation of curds in his stomach.

That person who likes watermelon first must know it is a natural cleanser that should be eaten at least two hours after a meal, or else before a meal.

And stale coffee's oils become rancid and harder to digest.

Let me throw my rules for better digestion at you. Better digestion means a better *you.* These rules are not all conclusive and they are probably more important for some people then for others. But they are tried and true and worth looking over and probably paying some mind to. They are in no special order — just random as they have come to me:

- Chew slowly and well, especially starches.
- Eat balanced meals, with complete proteins.
- Eat natural foods, replete with vitamins and minerals.
- Avoid processed and refined foods and limit sweets.
- Drink water freely between meals, but sparingly during meals.
- Cook with low heats; avoid frying.
- Cook vegetables minimally and use little water.
- Eat some raw fruits and raw vegetables every day.
- Limit condiments like salt, pepper, ketchup.
- Flavor foods with natural herbs and spices.
- Try to avoid eating between meals.
- Make your heavy meal mid-day, not evening.
- Limit tea and coffee and other stimulants.
- Favor organ meats. Avoid cold cuts.
- Avoid hydrogenated fats and oils.

Observed, each one of these fifteen principles will contribute to a high efficiency of digestion and every cell in your body will say, "Thank you."

THE BEST WAYS TO GET ESSENTIAL PROTEIN

Soybeans should not be eaten raw as they contain a toxic substance that is neutralized by cooking. Soy is an antacid and contains many vitamins and minerals. It can be worked into just about any kind of recipe from meat loaf to bread.

As the price of meat goes up, more and more people are leaning on plant proteins. But the picture needs to be complete, using all the jigsaw pieces — grains, legumes (peas, beans, etc.), vegetables, nuts, and seeds.

Some change in livestock feeding methods is taking place because of rising prices — for the better.

Our forefathers used to raise cattle by permitting them to forage, that is, to graze on grass, alfalfa, and clover in the pasture.

Later, stockmen found they could fatten up the animals faster by shipping them to a feedlot for six months prior to slaughter. Here they were fed on corn or sorghum. This is the fatter meat and more tender to which we have now grown accustomed.

However, the price of feed is so high, cattlemen are returning to the less expensive way of feeding their livestock. We are seeing leaner meat on the market and this means a greater percentage of protein, as the fat content is lowered.

Also, the lowered saturated fat content is surely going to mean fewer heart attacks and fewer circulatory problems for the population in general.

Higher prices can be a boon if they bring us back to natural ways.

Complete protein — lowered saturated fat. That's like a one, two punch for better health.

AN EASY WAY TO LOSE WEIGHT

Some people's drinking habits are as bad as their eating habits. I don't mean liquor. I mean water. Yes, liquor is abused. So are sweet drinks — soda pop. But even water is not imbibed sensibly.

If we drink before our stomach has completed digesting a meal, we dilute the stomach juices and interfere with digestion.

It requires approximately three and one-half hours for the stomach to empty after a meal. That is the period you should wait before taking liquids. It is far better to drink before a meal than during or after.

If fluid is taken during the digestive process, the body often accumulates the fluid. It is carried around as excess poundage. Sometimes this fluid accumulation is the result of faulty kidney, bowel, or perspiration action. But no matter what it is due to, it adds up to excess pounds and inches.

Excess fluid is one of the causes of obesity. Where it is present, there is a simple way to lose weight: Stop drinking water and other liquids during and after meals.

Try this: Wait three and a half hours after each meal before drinking liquids. Weigh and measure the difference in one week.

Take the case of Mrs. Rene C. in her early 20's. She was pleasingly plump, having acquired her excess pounds gradually over a period of two years. She said dieting did not help.

She was instructed to stop drinking liquids for at least three and one-half hours after each meal. After faithfully following this method for two weeks, she had lost a total of fourteen pounds. Needless to say, she was more than pleased with herself and commented that she no longer had "that logy, tired feeling." No diet or other plan for weight reduction was followed other than the liquid restriction during the two weeks. She ate at the usual times, the usual fare, and the usual quantities. But still she lost unusually fast. Her body let go of that stored up fluid and she did not permit any more to take its place.

Carrying around excess baggage is a load on the heart and other organs. We talk a lot about growing old gracefully, but it's more like grossfully. Older people need to watch their fluid intake and their weight with increasing vigilance.

YOU CAN TALK YOURSELF INTO BETTER HEALTH

If you were permitted to eavesdrop when the old family doctor was treating a patient, you would hear a lot of talking going on. It would be about business, town happenings, family situations. It often sounded like a social visit. But don't mistake it — important therapy was taking place.

The family doctor was interested in each patient as a person. That person's life was part of his condition. So he not only took the pulse of his heart, but the pulse of his times. He examined the whole person.

A recent John Hopkins Hospital survey found that three out of four illnesses were psychosomatic. That is, they were caused by emotional factors. This does not mean that the pain in the head was imaginary, or that the pain in the stomach was not real.

A psychosomatic illness is like any other illness. In fact, it *is* any other illness. Major events in our life cause emotional reactions which in turn are accompanied by biochemical changes that can put our metabolic processes out of balance. That spells disease. Not imagined. Very real, painful disease.

Fear, excitement, strain — all weaken the body's immunity and upset hormone production.

When a patient tells his doctor about these matters, it relieves the fear or stress. It gets it off his chest. The body responds.

A game that is played in modern human potential groups is called "Doctor — Patient." The participants pair off and take turns playing doctor. All the "doctors" do is listen to their "patients'" problems. Participants unload their tensions. They feel good because their body loves it.

Many medical men are coming around to the realization that just about every sickness or disease can have its root cause in some attitudes or emotions which interfere with the body's defenses or balances.

Even a disease as difficult to find a cure for as cancer is now being studied for psychosomatic causes. Recently a task force of the American Psychological Association has summarized these studies which find that certain personality traits may predispose a person to cancer. These include a repressive personality pattern; a tendency to respond to a loss with hopelessness or despair; and a personality that is tense, defensive, and anxious.

The age of specialization made specialists in the heart, the lungs, the throat, and other organs. The old-time family doctor specialized in people. He looked at the whole person — his mind, personality, troubles, family.

We may be coming back to that.

Stress, according to a University of Rochester study, is the cause behind most physical illnesses. Emotional stress that leads a person to an attitude of "I give up" or "I can't take it anymore" is tantamount to giving the body instructions to get sick.

People with certain character traits get sick in the same places or ways. It can manifest as arthritis for one kind of personality, skin condition for another.

Talking about your problems is one way to externalize the situation. You take it outside of your body and release it. You virtually unload your stress on somebody else.

If that somebody else is you, be careful you do not take the problem on yourself. Be objective. Don't be too sympathetic to the extent that you put yourself in the troubled person's shoes.

WALK AWAY FROM HEALTH PROBLEMS

Talking helps. So does walking. I have already discussed walking as a remedy for certain conditions. Besides a general health stimulant, walking can help with such specific problems as constipation, chronic diarrhea, bladder incontinence. Arterial pumping becomes more vigorous and effective. The flow of lymphatic and venous fluids is accelerated the better to refine out impurities and metabolic byproducts. Walking is like taking an internal bath.

But walking is something else. It is also a mental bath. Sights and sounds change. Your thoughts go to other matters than the ones that are bugging you. Your lungs take in fresh air along with the fresh thoughts. You see things in a new perspective. Probably you have left your walls and a ceiling behind and are now getting a larger range view of the world.

So besides being a physical boon to your body by the stimulation the motion of walking provides, it is also a mental boon to your body — and that corrects and removes the cause of illness.

When you walk away from a troubled situation out into the fresh air, you are literally walking away from illness.

HOW TO ORDER YOUR BODY TO BEHAVE

A branch of medicine is now making strides in helping people to help themselves out of physical problems — especially when the emotional cause of those problems is apparent.

The technique they use is called suggestive therapy. It works when you believe in it. It does not work if you don't. The mind obeys your instructions. If you say "I believe this," you are instructing the mind to cooperate. If you say, "This is not for me," you are telling the mind not to cooperate.

The mind obeys in either case.

The mind obeys this and it also obeys what follows — suggestions or commands to change the way it is operating your body — changes for the better, of course.

You can induce ulcers to heal.

You can lower your blood pressure.

You can "command" headaches to end.

The trick is to relax and get very peaceful before giving the body the instructions you want it to follow. This relaxation permits the command to get through to the automatic part of your brain which controls your body's operation.

Another trick is to add a mental picture to the words. In other words, besides commanding ulcers to heal, see your stomach lining free of any sores. Use your imagination — the imagining mind seems to have a direct wire to the automatic mind and its pictures act as powerful instructions.

Here is the secret of how to relax. Lie in a comfortable position. Close your eyes. Command your toes to relax as you visualize them. Next ankles, calves, knees, etc. Relax the entire body, part by part this way. Then you are ready to give corrective suggestions or commands directed at whatever physical problem you wish to correct.

New? Not on your life. It goes back to ancient days. And it still works "miracles."

Miss S., age 40, had been an asthmatic most of her life. In consultation I had found that she had certain experiences that triggered off the inability to bring adequate air into her lungs. These were experiences that the average person would not give a second thought to, but which were emotionally unpleasant to her and would cause her to choke up. At these times, if she did not use her medication, she could develop a severe asthmatic attack.

She told me she did not like to have to resort to using the medication, but she did not care to have the asthmatic attack, either. I did not discourage her from using her medication. However, I told her the next time she had one of her "bad experiences" to calmly sit down and to concentrate on relaxing her lungs, bronchi, rib cage, in fact, her entire respiratory system. I told her she would get out of this exercise as much relaxation as she put concentration into it.

A month later Miss S. returned to my office telling me that she had not had to resort to her medication for almost thirty days. She'd had three of her bad experiences, but she had done exactly as I had instructed, and felt immediate relaxation in her breathing.

We keep giving ourselves suggestions all the time. My mother used to think cherry pie would make you sick. She always got sick from eating cherry pie. Her body obeyed her mind.

We keep saying things like "I can't see that" or "He gives me a pain in the neck" or "That burns me up" — ordering: one case of myopia with a stiff neck and a fever to go with it.

Avoid destructive, negative statements and thoughts. See the glass half full, not half empty. Realize that everything that happens can be made to happen for the best, and behind the darkest cloud is a beautiful sunlit sky.

THE FUEL THAT MAKES YOUR BODY RUN AT ITS BEST

A doctor being interviewed on the radio was asked how to get rid of a common cold. His answer was, "Fall in love."

This may sound like an unusual prescription, but try it. The happiness and exalted feeling of love stimulates the entire body to more perfect functioning.

Actually, falling in love is just one way to attain this. The chief ingredient of love is in many other facets of life — it is called enthusiasm.

The sick person with no enthusiasm for life is a goner. Doctors recognize that an enthusiastic desire to live is the best medicine for healthy people, too. In fact, it is the fuel that powers us.

A person without enthusiasm is a negative person. Such a person is prone to inertia. No get up and go. Inert means totally unreactive.

I have seen people who are inert. They are in the doldrums. They "have the misery." They get into one state of sickness after another. Medicines may cure one condition, but their lack of enthusiasm sinks them right back into another condition.

One young depressed woman had a fever for weeks. Nothing helped. Then her boyfriend called. She perked up right away and down went the fever.

This is a great life. It is so great there is little room for improvement on nature. We are all children of nature, born to be perfect, to live life in our own unique way — naturally.

Rejoice in nature. Live with enthusiasm. And claim your heritage — good health.

INDEX